APPLE CIDER VINEGAR

Heal · cleanse · rejuvenate

Publications International, Ltd.

Photography for the front cover and page 4 by Christopher Hiltz

Photo styling by Stephanie Rocha

Additional images from Shutterstock.com

Louis Weber, CEO
Publications International, Ltd.
8140 Lehigh Avenue
Morton Grove, IL 60053

Permission is never granted for commercial purposes.

ISBN: 978-1-64030-157-3

Manufactured in China.

8 7 6 5 4 3 2 1

Note: Neither the editors of Publications International, Ltd., nor the authors, consultants, editors, or publisher take responsibility for any possible consequence from any treatment, procedure, exercise, dietary modification, action, or application of medication or preparation by any person reading or following the information in this book. The publication of this book does not constitute the practice of medicine, and this book does not attempt to replace your physician or your pharmacist. Before undertaking any course of treatment, the authors, consultants, editors, and publisher advise the reader to check with a physician or other health care provider.

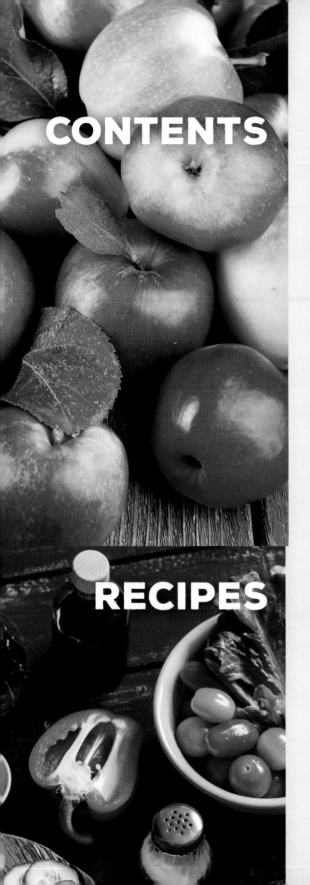

CONTENTS

RECIPES

INTRODUCTION

If you were told that there was a new product on the market that could act as a general remedy and tonic, ease aches, soothe skin ailments, help with colds and headaches, tone your face, condition your hair, help clean your household, add flavor to meals, and even lower your blood sugar, you'd probably be skeptical. How could one substance do all those things? But age-old vinegar serves all those purposes. In its various forms, vinegar can be a healer, a disinfectant, a preservative, an acid, and a condiment. This list is pretty impressive considering vinegar is a byproduct of something gone bad!

Apple cider vinegar has long been a popular folk remedy. These days, it is coming back into its own, and people are discovering additional health benefits. While it's not a miracle cure, it can play a role in a healthy diet, crucial to maintaining good health. In this book we'll explore some of apple cider vinegar's many uses. We'll also offer guidance for creating your own home remedies using apple cider vinegar, as well as delicious food recipes.

In chapter 1, Vinegar Basics, you'll learn about how vinegar is made—and even how to make your own apple cider vinegar! While we focus on apple cider vinegar in this book, many varieties of vinegar offer health benefits, so this chapter offers a quick over-view of the different kinds of vinegars, as well as ideas for adding herbs to vinegars to create wonderful flavor combinations.

Chapter 2, Apple Cider Vinegar Remedies, provides an assortment of remedies drawn from folk traditions, to address common conditions including aches and sore muscles, athlete's foot, itching from poison ivy, the common cold, foot pain, stomach upset, and more.

Chapter 3, Body and Hair Care, shows how apple cider vinegar can be used as a facial toner and hair conditioner. Whether your skin and hair are oily or dry, you'll find facial splashes and herbal rinses to help you out.

While vinegar can help you out personally, it can also help out your household! Explore some of those uses in chapter 4, Pet Care, and chapter 5, Home and Garden Care.

Chapter 6, The Benefits of Vinegar in Your Diet, looks at some of the ways vinegar can help your body in the long term, by controlling blood sugar, replacing fats, and more.

Vinegar can be paired with other substances, such as herbs and essential oils, for increased health benefits. In chapter 7, Herbs and Vinegar, we'll look at some of the healing benefits of herbs commonly paired with vinegar. In chapter 8, Aromatherapy and Essential Oils, we'll examine some oils for which vinegar can act as a "carrier oil," and offer some home remedies involving essential oils for sunburn, fungal infections, and poison ivy.

The last section of the book includes recipes that use apple cider vinegar—and a few other tasty vinegar varieties. From salad vinaigrettes to wholesome main meals, you'll find dozens of delicious recipes.

From body care to ingredient, remedy to carrier oil, apple cider vinegar has a number of amazing uses. So make apple cider vinegar a part of your diet and your life—you'll be glad you did!

Throughout the book, when directed to make a paste, mix a dry ingredient with a liquid ingredient to the consistency of tootpaste. Exact measurements are unimportant.

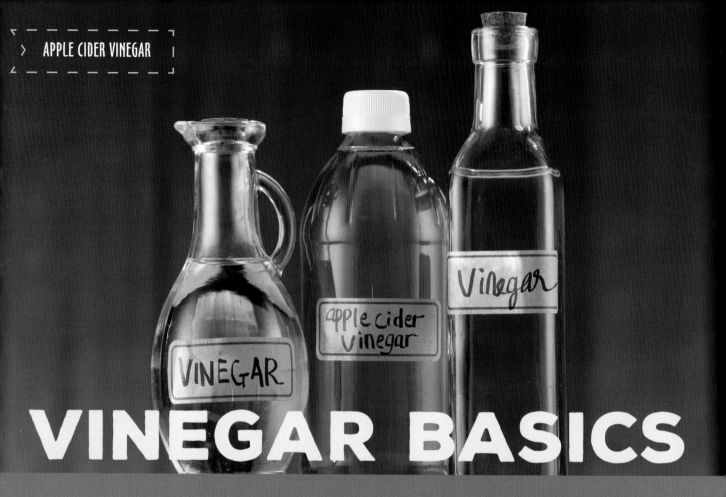

VINEGAR BASICS

JUST WHAT IS VINEGAR?

Vinegar is a dilute solution of acetic acid that results from a two-step fermentation process. The first step is the fermentation of sugar into alcohol, usually by yeast. Any natural source of sugar can be used. For example, the sugar may be derived from the juice, or cider, of fruit (such as grapes, apples, raisins, or even coconuts); from a grain (such as barley or rice); from honey, molasses, or sugar cane; or even, in the case of certain distilled vinegars, from the cellulose in wood (such as beech).

What you have at the end of this first phase, then, is an alcohol-containing liquid, such as wine (from grapes), beer (from barley), hard cider (from apples), or another fermented liquid. The alcoholic liquid used to create a vinegar is generally reflected in the vinegar's name—for example, red wine vinegar, white wine vinegar, malt vinegar, or cider vinegar.

In the second phase of the vinegar-production process, certain naturally occurring bacteria known as acetobacters combine the alcohol-containing liquid with oxygen to form the acetic-acid solution we call vinegar. Acetic acid is what gives vinegar its sour taste. Although time-consuming, this second phase of the process will happen without human intervention if the alcoholic liquid is exposed to oxygen long enough.

ALL ABOUT ACIDITY

The U.S. Food and Drug Administration requires that vinegar contain a minimum of 4 percent acetic acid. White vinegar is typically 5 percent acetic acid, and cider and wine vinegars are a bit more acidic, usually between 5 percent and 6 percent. A little acidity goes a long way—acetic acid is in fact corrosive and can destroy living tissues when concentrated. An acetic acid level of 11 percent or more can burn the skin. And according to the Consumer Product Safety Commission, an "acetic acid preparation containing free or chemically unneutralized acetic acid in a concentration of 20 percent or more" is considered poison. In fact, a 20 percent acetic acid concentration is sometimes used as an herbicide to kill garden weeds.

> The bloodstream of a healthy adult has a pH that is mildly alkaline—about 7.41. Vinegar is a strongly acidic solution with a pH of around 2.

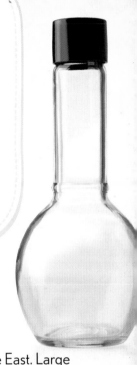

THE HISTORY OF VINEGAR

The first vinegar was the result of an ancient, serendipitous, accident. Once upon a time, a keg of wine (presumably a poorly sealed one that allowed oxygen in) was stored too long, and when the would-be drinkers opened it, they found a sour liquid instead of wine. The name "vinegar" is derived from the French words for "sour wine."

Fortunately, our resourceful ancestors found ways to use the "bad" wine. They put it to work as a cure-all, a food preservative, and later, a flavor enhancer. It wasn't long before they figured out how to make vinegar on purpose, and producing it became one of the world's earliest commercial industries.

Scientists believe wine originated during the Neolithic period (approximately 8500 B.C. to 4000 B.C., when humans first began farming and crafting stone tools) in Egypt and the Middle East. Large pottery jugs dating back to 6000 B.C. that were unearthed in archaeological digs possessed a strange yellow residue. Chemical analysis revealed the residue contained calcium tartrate, which is formed from tartaric acid, a substance that occurs naturally in large amounts only in grapes. So the traces strongly suggest the jugs were used to make or hold wine.

Considering the slow grape-pressing methods used at that time and the heat of the desert environment, grape juice would likely have fermented into wine quite quickly. Likewise, the wine would have turned to vinegar rapidly, if conditions were right.

So how did these ancient people—who had only recently (in evolutionary terms) begun planting their

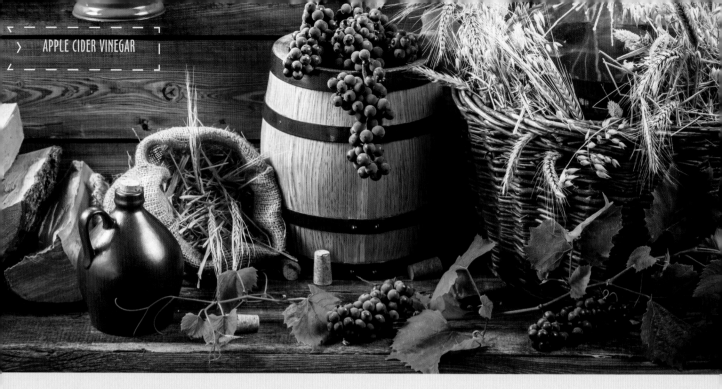

own food and fashioning tools—manage to understand and control fermentation enough to prevent all their wine from turning to vinegar before they could drink it? Based on evidence found in archaeological excavations, scientists believe that the first winemakers used jars with clay stoppers that helped control the fermentation process.

A complete analysis of the residue left in those ancient wine jugs also showed the presence of terebinth tree resin, which acts as a natural preservative and therefore would have helped slow the transformation of wine into vinegar. In Neolithic times, terebinth trees grew in the same area as grapes, and their berries and resin were harvested at the same time of year. So it's quite plausible that some of the berries or resins may have inadvertently become mixed with the grape harvest. Still unclear is whether the ancient winemakers ever made the connection between the resins and the delayed conversion of wine into vinegar and began purposely adding the tree berries to their wine.

Throughout the world there are only 12 copies of something known as The Vinegar Bible, a version of the Christian Bible printed in 1717. The edition features beautiful engravings and elegant type. However, it also contains numerous typos, including a misuse of the word vinegar. In the New Testament's parable of the vineyard, the heading reads, "The parable of the vinegar."

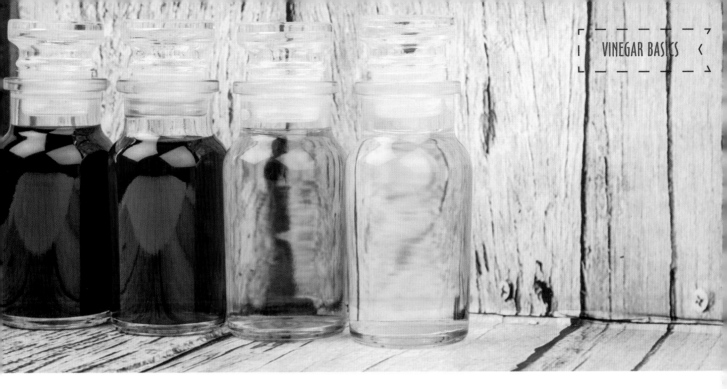

VINEGAR VARIETIES

You might be surprised to learn that there are dozens of types of vinegar. The most common vinegars found in American kitchens are white distilled and apple cider, but the more adventurous may also use red wine vinegar, white wine vinegar, rice vinegar, or gourmet varieties, such as 25-year-old balsamic vinegar or rich black fig vinegar.

As you've learned, vinegar can be made from just about any food that contains natural sugars. Yeast ferments these sugars into alcohol, and certain types of bacteria convert that alcohol a second time into vinegar. A weak acetic acid remains after this second fermentation; the acid has flavors reminiscent of the original fermented food, such as apples or grapes. Acetic acid is what gives vinegar its distinct tart taste.

Pure acetic acid can be made in a laboratory; when diluted with water, it is sometimes sold as white vinegar. However, acetic acids created in labs lack the subtle flavors found in true vinegars, and synthesized versions don't hold a candle to vinegars fermented naturally from summer's sugar-laden fruits or from other foods.

Vinegars can be made from many different foods that add their own tastes to the final products, but additional ingredients, such as herbs, spices, or fruits, can be added for further flavor enhancement. For more about that, see page 14.

Vinegar is great for a healthy, light style of cooking. The tangy taste often reduces the need for salt, especially in soups and bean dishes. It can also cut the fat in a recipe because it balances flavors without requiring the addition of as much cream, butter, or oil. Vinegar flavors range from mild to bold, so you're sure to find one with the taste you want. A brief look at some of the various vinegars available may help you choose a new one for your culinary escapades.

WHITE VINEGAR

This clear variety is the most common type of vinegar in American households. It is made either from grain-based ethanol or laboratory-produced acetic acid and then diluted with water. Its flavor is a bit too harsh for most cooking uses, but it is good for pickling and performing many cleaning jobs around the house. For more about cleaning, see Home and Garden Care on pages 56–57.

APPLE CIDER VINEGAR

Apple cider vinegar is the second-most-common type of vinegar in the United States. This light-tan vinegar made from apple cider adds a tart and subtle fruity flavor to your cooking. Along with its health uses, apple cider vinegar is best for salads, dressings, marinades, condiments, and most general vinegar needs.

WINE VINEGAR

This flavorful type of vinegar is made from a blend of either red wines or white wines and is common in Europe, especially Germany. Creative cooks often infuse wine vinegars with extra flavor by tucking in a few sprigs of well-washed fresh herbs, dried herbs, or fresh berries. Red wine vinegar is often flavored with natural raspberry flavoring, if not with the fruit itself.

The quality of the original wine determines how good the vinegar is. Better wine vinegars are made from good wines and are aged for a couple of years or more in wooden casks. The result is a fuller, more complex, and mellow flavor.

You might find sherry vinegar on the shelf next to the wine vinegars. This variety is made from sherry wine and is usually imported from Spain. Champagne vinegar (yes, made from the bubbly stuff) is a specialty vinegar and is quite expensive.

Wine vinegar excels at bringing out the sweetness of fruit, melon, and berries and adds a flavorful punch to fresh salsa.

BALSAMIC VINEGAR

There are two types of this popular and delicious vinegar, traditional and commercial. A quasi-governmental body in Modena, Italy (balsamic vinegar's birthplace), regulates the production of traditional balsamic vinegar.

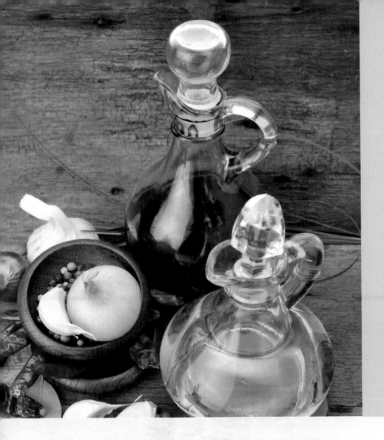

You might see that some traditional balsamic vinegars have leaves on their labels. This is a rating system that ranks quality on a one- to four-leaf scale, with four leaves being the best. You can use the leaf ranking as a guide for how to use the vinegar. For instance, one-leaf balsamic vinegar would be appropriate for salad dressing, while four-leaf vinegar would be best used a few drops at a time to season a dish right before serving. The Assaggiatori Italiani Balsamico (Italian Balsamic Tasters' Association) established this grading system, but not all producers use it.

TRADITIONAL BALSAMIC

Traditional balsamic vinegars are artisanal foods, similar to great wines, with long histories and well-developed customs for their production. An excellent balsamic vinegar can be made only by an experienced crafter who has spent many years tending the vinegar, patiently watching and learning.

The luscious white and sugary trebbiano grapes that are grown in the northern region of Italy near Modena form the base of the world's best and only true balsamic vinegars. Custom dictates that the grapes be left on the vine for as long as possible to develop their sugar. The juice (or "must") is pressed out of the grapes and boiled down; then, vinegar production begins.

Traditional balsamic vinegar is aged for a number of years—typically 6 and as many as 25. Aging takes place in a succession of casks made from a variety of woods, such as chestnut, mulberry, oak, juniper, and cherry. Each producer has its own formula for the order in which the vinegar is moved to the different casks. Thus, the flavors are complex, rich, sweet, and subtly woody. Vinegar made in this way carries a seal from the Consortium of Producers of the Traditional Balsamic Vinegar of Modena.

Because of the arduous production process, only a limited amount of traditional balsamic vinegar makes it to market each year, and what is available is expensive.

COMMERCIAL BALSAMIC

What you're more likely to find in most American grocery stores is the commercial type of balsamic vinegar. Some is made in Modena, but not by traditional methods. In fact, some balsamic vinegar isn't even made in Italy. Commercial balsamic vinegar does not carry the Consortium of Producers of the Traditional Balsamic Vinegar of Modena seal because it is not produced in accordance with the Consortium's strict regulations.

The production of commercial balsamic vinegar carries no geographical restrictions or rules for length or method of aging. There are no requirements for the types of wood used in the aging casks. It may be aged for six months in stainless steel vats, then for two years or more in wood. Thus, commercial balsamic vinegar is much more affordable and available than the true, artisanal variety.

Whether you're lucky enough to get your hands on the traditional variety or you're using commercial-grade balsamic, the taste of this fine vinegar is like no other. Its sweet and sour notes are in perfect proportion. Balsamic's flavor is so intricate that it brings out the best in salty foods such as goat cheese, astringent foods such as spinach, and sweet foods such as strawberries.

RICE VINEGAR

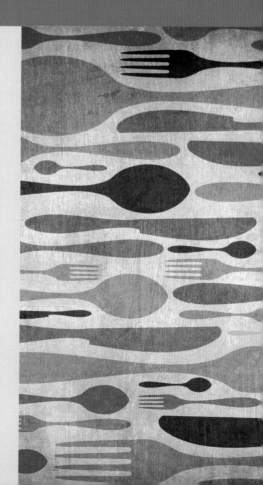

Clear or very pale yellow, rice vinegar originated in Japan, where it is essential to sushi preparation. Rice vinegar is made from the sugars found in rice, and the aged, filtered final product has a mild, clean, and delicate flavor that is an excellent complement to ginger or cloves, sometimes with the addition of sugar.

Rice vinegar also comes in red and black varieties, which are not common in the United States but very popular in China. Both are stronger than the clear (often called white) or pale yellow types. Red rice vinegar's flavor is a combination of sweet and tart. Black rice vinegar is common in southern Chinese cooking and has a strong, almost smoky flavor. Rice vinegar is popular in Asian cooking and is great sprinkled on salads and stir-fry dishes. Its gentle flavor is perfect for fruits and tender vegetables, too. Many cooks choose white rice vinegar for their recipes because it does not change the color of the food to which it is added. Red rice vinegar is good for soups and noodle dishes, and black rice vinegar works as a dipping sauce and in braised dishes.

MALT VINEGAR

This dark-brown vinegar, a favorite in Britain, is reminiscent of deep-brown ale. Malt vinegar production begins with the germination, or sprouting, of barley kernels. Germination enables enzymes to break down starch into sugar. The resulting product is brewed into an alcohol-containing malt beverage or ale. After bacteria convert the ale to vinegar, the vinegar is aged. As its name implies, malt vinegar has a distinctive malt flavor. A cheaper and less flavorful version of malt vinegar consists merely of acetic acid diluted to between 4 percent and 8 percent acidity, with a little caramel coloring added.

Many people prefer malt vinegar for pickling and as an accompaniment to fish and chips. It is also used as the basic type of cooking vinegar in Britain.

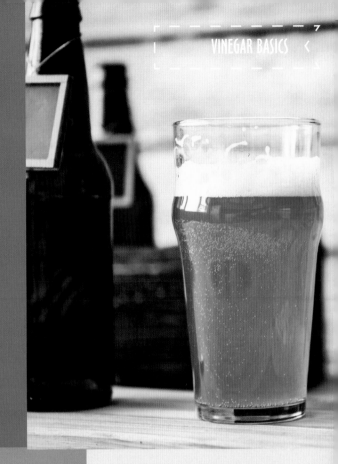

COCONUT VINEGAR

If you can't get your Asian recipes to taste "just right," it might be because you don't have coconut vinegar—a white vinegar with a sharp, acidic, slightly yeasty taste. This staple of Southeast Asian cooking is made from the sap of the coconut palm and is especially important to Thai and Indian dishes.

CANE VINEGAR

This type of vinegar is produced from the sugar cane and is used mainly in the Philippines. It is often light yellow and has a flavor similar to rice vinegar. Contrary to what you might think, cane vinegar is not any sweeter than other vinegars.

BEER VINEGAR

Beer vinegar has an appealing light-golden color and, as you might guess, is popular in Germany, Austria, Bavaria, and the Netherlands. It is made from beer, and its flavor depends on the brew from which it was made.

RAISIN VINEGAR

This slightly cloudy, brown vinegar is traditionally produced in Turkey and used in Middle Eastern cuisines. Try infusing it with a little cinnamon to bolster its mild flavor. Salad dressings made with raisin vinegar will add an unconventional taste to your greens.

PASTEURIZED FOR YOUR PROTECTION

Some apple cider vinegars proudly proclaim to be "raw, organic, and unpasteurized," but beware: Buying an unpasteurized product is risky business.

Most apple cider is made from apples that have fallen to the ground, and the bacterium *E. coli* can easily contaminate these fruits. If processors don't wash off this deadly bacterium before the apples are pressed, and the final product is not pasteurized, there is a risk of *E. coli* contamination, which can lead to severe health problems and even death.

Although most bacteria cannot survive in the acidic conditions of vinegar, the acidity of the unpasteurized product can weaken over time, thus allowing bacteria to grow—and making the product dangerous for you. To be on the safe side, be sure you always choose vinegars that have been prepared, pasteurized, and stored properly.

HERBS AND VINEGAR

Whether you start with homemade or store-bought vinegar, you can kick it up by adding flavorful herbs or spices. This also helps you preserve your homegrown herbs! You can use your herbal vinegar in nearly any recipe that calls for plain vinegar.

Add herb leaves or seeds to white vinegar or apple cider vinegar. Garlic, basil, rosemary, and tarragon are herbs commonly added to white wine vinegar. Cider vinegar is recommended for some of the stronger herbs such as dill, garlic, garlic chives, and horseradish. Balsamic vinegar or vinegar made with sherry or champagne is best for preserving oregano. Other herbs or fruits, such as raspberries, also can enhance vinegar's taste. These additions leave their flavors and trace amounts of healthy nutrients, too.

Use ½ cup to 1 cup freshly crushed or bruised herb leaves to every 2 cups vinegar. The vinegar must completely cover the leaves. Store mixture in a sealed, nonmetal container (metal will react with the vinegar), and let it sit in a cool, dark place. Sample vinegar after a week to see if the flavor is as you would like. After 4 weeks, you will have extracted all the possible flavor out of the herb. Pour vinegar into decorative bottles with caps or cork stoppers. Unopened, the flavored vinegar will last up to 2 years. Opened, it will last 3 to 6 months.

Herbal vinegars need to be carefully prepared to avoid contamination with potentially harmful bacteria. Most bacteria cannot exist in vinegar's acidic environment, but a few deadly ones can, so follow these basic steps:

- Use only high-quality vinegars when creating flavor combinations.

- Remember that red and white wine vinegar, though great for flavoring, contain trace amounts of protein that could give harmful bacteria an ideal place to live unless you prepare and store the vinegars properly.

- Wash your storage bottles and then sterilize them by completely immersing them in boiling water for 10 minutes. Always fill the bottles while they are still warm, and be sure you have a tight-fitting lid, cap, or cork for each one.

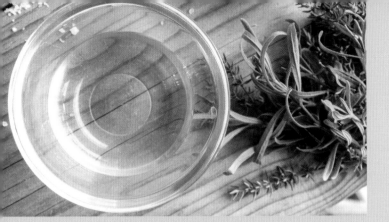

• If you're using fresh herbs, there is a risk of harmful bacteria hitchhiking their way into the vinegar via the sprigs. Commercial vinegar processors use antimicrobial agents to sanitize herbs, but you probably won't be able to find these chemicals. University extension publications recommend mixing one teaspoon of bleach into six cups of water and dipping the fresh herbs into this solution. Then rinse the herbs thoroughly and pat them dry. This will minimize the possibility of any harmful bacteria making their way into the vinegar and will not affect the taste.

• Be sure your fresh herbs are in top-notch condition—bruising or decay indicates the presence of bacteria. If you harvest your own herbs, do so in the morning, when the essential oils are at their peak.

• Mix it up a bit by adding some spices or vegetables, such as garlic or hot peppers. Thread garlic, peppers, or other small items on a skewer so you can remove them easily when you've infused enough flavor.

• To add fruit flavors to vinegar, thoroughly wash fruit, berries, or citrus rind. Use one to two cups of fruit for every pint of vinegar, but only the rind of one lemon or orange per pint. You can thread small fruits or chunks of fruit on a skewer and tie chopped rind in a small piece of clean cheesecloth to make removal easy.

• When you're ready to start mixing, place the herbs or flavoring in the sterilized, hot bottles. Heat the vinegar to 190 degrees Fahrenheit and then pour it over the herbs in the sterilized bottles. Heating the vinegar to 190 degrees Fahrenheit will prevent bacteria from forming and also help release the essential oils from the herbs, spices, or fruits.

• Put a tight-fitting lid on your container and allow the vinegar to stand in a cool, dark place for three to four weeks. When it has enough flavor, strain it through a cheesecloth or coffee filter several times until any cloudiness is gone.

• Discard the fruits, spices, or herbs and pour the filtered vinegar into newly sterilized containers. If you want to add a decorative herb sprig, sanitize it first.

• Store the vinegar in the refrigerator for the best flavor retention; it will keep well for six to eight months. Unrefrigerated vinegar will keep its flavor for only two to three months. If the bottle has been left to look pretty on a sunny windowsill for more than a few weeks, use the vinegar only as decoration, not as food.

For more about herbs and vinegar, see pages 72–86.

CHILI VINEGAR

Put 3 ounces chopped chilies into 1 quart vinegar, and store for 2 weeks in a capped bottle. Strain liquid after 2 weeks. For a spicier, stronger vinegar, let chilies steep longer, to taste.

GARLIC VINEGAR

Peel cloves from 1 large bulb of garlic, and add them to 1 quart vinegar. Steep liquid for 2 weeks, then strain and discard garlic. Use a few drops for flavoring salads, cooked meat, or vegetables. Variation: Use 1 quart red wine vinegar for a resulting vinegar that can be used in place of fresh garlic in most recipes. One teaspoon of the garlic vinegar will be equivalent to a small clove of garlic.

STRAWBERRY VINEGAR

Combine a bottle of white wine vinegar with 1/2 cup fresh, washed, and stemmed strawberries. Cover and let it sit at room temperature for 1 week. Remove fruit, and use vinegar in recipes calling for fruit vinegar, or sprinkle on a lettuce salad.

CUCUMBER-ONION VINEGAR

Boil 1 pint vinegar, and add 1 teaspoon salt and a dash of white pepper. Add 2 sliced pickling cucumbers and 1 small onion, sliced very thin, to vinegar mixture. Store in a capped glass jar for 5 weeks, then strain. Pour strained liquid into a recycled wine bottle, and cork it. Variation: Leave out onion for a very light vinegar that's excellent on fruit salads.

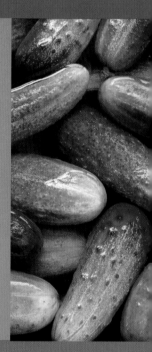

HOT PEPPER VINEGAR

Pour 1 pint vinegar into a clean bottle with cap, then add 1/2 ounce cayenne pepper to it. Let mixture sit for 2 weeks out of direct sunlight. Shake bottle about every other day. After 2 weeks, strain and pour into a separate clean bottle for use.

RASPBERRY VINEGAR

Make a raspberry vinegar with 2 quarts water and 5 quarts red or black raspberries. Pour water over 1 quart washed red or black raspberries, and keep in airtight container. Let stand over-night, then strain and keep liquid (discard raspberries). Pour liquid over another quart of raspberries, then strain and discard raspberries. Add 1 pound sugar to strained liquid, and stir until dissolved. Let mixture stand uncovered for 2 months, strain, then use as vinegar.

MAKE YOUR OWN APPLE CIDER VINEGAR

You can not only add herbs to vinegar for better flavors—you can even make your own vinegar! Experimenting with flavors can be fun, and it's especially rewarding to use your own vinegar in your favorite dishes or to give it as a gift.

You'll want to get exact directions from your local brewing supply store or university extension service. Be sure the directions you follow are tested and researched for safety to avoid food-borne illness. Take a look at this rundown of the general process to make apple cider vinegar to see if you're up to the task:

• Make apple cider by pressing clean, washed, ripe apples (fall apples have more sugar than early-season apples). Strain to make a clean juice and pour it into sterilized containers.

• Use yeast designed for brewing wine or beer (not baker's yeast) to ferment the fruit sugar into alcohol.

• Now let bacteria convert the alcohol to acetic acid. Leaving the fermenting liquid uncovered invites acid-making bacteria to take up residence. (You might, however, want to place some cheesecloth or a towel over your container's opening to prevent insects, dirt, or other nasty items from getting into the mixture.) Some vinegar brewers use a "mother of vinegar" (see sidebar) as a "starter," or source of the acid-producing bacteria.

If you see a jellylike cloudy film collecting in the bottom of your vinegar bottle, you've discovered the "mother of vinegar." It's merely cellulose made by acid-producing bacteria. Mother of vinegar is a completely natural by-product of vinegar that contains live bacteria. It is harmless and is not a sign of contamination. Just strain off the liquid vinegar and continue using it. Most manufacturers pasteurize their vinegar to prevent mother of vinegar from forming. Some say this goo prevents infectious diseases if you eat a little each day, but there is no research to verify that belief.

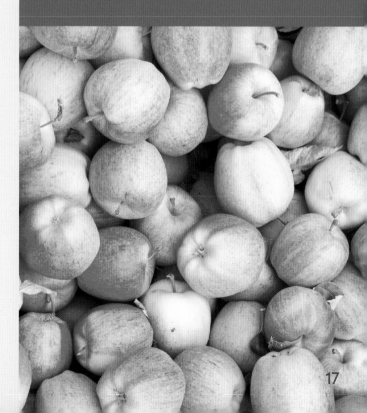

• Keep the liquid between 60 degrees and 80 degrees Fahrenheit during the fermentation process; it will take three to four weeks to make vinegar. If you keep the liquid too cool, the vinegar may be unusable. If it's kept too warm, it may not form the mother of vinegar mat at the bottom of the container. The mother of vinegar mat signifies proper fermentation.

• Stir the liquid daily to introduce adequate amounts of oxygen, which is necessary for fermentation.

• After three to four weeks, the bacteria will have converted most of the alcohol, and the mixture will begin to smell like vinegar. Taste a little bit each day until it reaches a flavor and acidity that you like.

• Strain the liquid through a cheesecloth or coffee filter several times to remove the mother of vinegar. Otherwise the fermentation process will continue and eventually spoil your vinegar.

• Store in sterilized, capped jars in the refrigerator.

• If you want to store homemade vinegar at room temperature for more than a few months, you must pasteurize it. Do this by heating it to 170 degrees Fahrenheit (use a cooking thermometer to determine the temperature) and hold it at this temperature for 10 minutes. Put the pasteurized vinegar in sterilized containers with tight-fitting lids, out of direct sunlight.

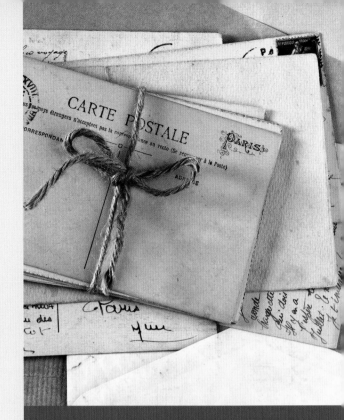

By the mid-1800s, greeting cards were enormously popular in Europe, inexpensive to create and send, and an important keepsake for the recipient. The notable exception to that paper happiness was the Penny Dreadful Valentine card, which cost one cent—also known as Vinegar Valentines. As the name implies, these cards were sour: The pictures and verse were insulting, and the cards were generally delivered to someone the sender disliked. Penny Dreadfuls were (un)popular starting in the 1850s.

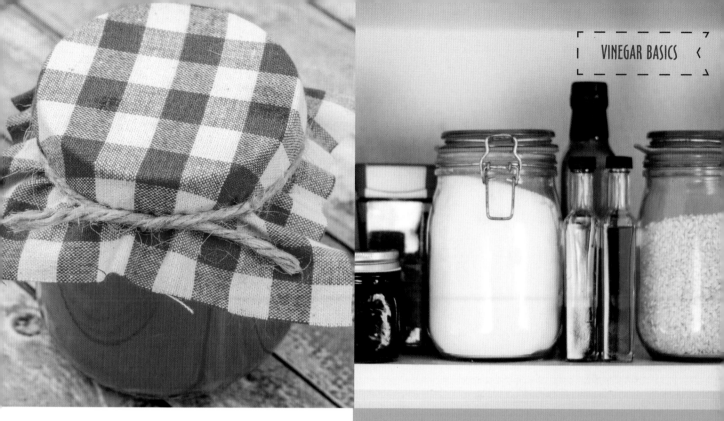

A HOMEMADE VINEGAR CAUTION

The acidity of homemade vinegar varies greatly. If you make your own vinegar, do not use it for canning, for preserving, or for anything that will be stored at room temperature. The vinegar's acidity, or pH level, may not be sufficient to preserve your food and could result in severe food poisoning. The pH level in homemade vinegar can weaken and allow pathogens, such as the deadly *E. coli,* to grow. Homemade vinegar is well suited for dressings, marinades, cooking, or pickled products that are stored in the refrigerator at all times.

VINEGAR STORAGE

Storing vinegar properly will hold flavor at its peak. Due to their high acid content, commercially prepared vinegars will keep almost indefinitely, even at room temperature. White vinegar will maintain its color, but other kinds may develop an off color or a haze. Neither of these conditions is a sign of spoilage; the vinegar is still good to use.

Store all vinegars in bottles sealed with airtight lids. Keep in a dark, cool place, and avoid direct sunlight, which can diminish flavor, color, and acidity. Homemade vinegars, especially herbal ones, are best stored in the refrigerator.

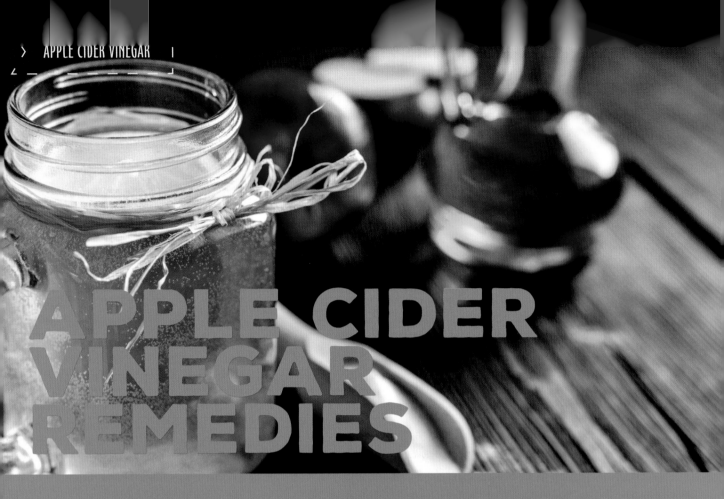

APPLE CIDER VINEGAR REMEDIES

The use of vinegar as medicine probably started soon after it was discovered. Its healing virtues are extolled in records of the Babylonians, and the great Greek physician Hippocrates reportedly used it as an antibiotic. Ancient Greek doctors poured vinegar into wounds and over dressings as a disinfectant, and they gave concoctions of honey and vinegar to patients recovering from illness. In Asia, early samurai warriors believed vinegar to be a tonic that would increase their strength and vitality.

Vinegar has continued to be used as a medicine in more recent times. During the Civil War and World War I, for example, military medics used vinegar to treat wounds. Folk traditions around the world still espouse vinegar for a wide variety of ailments. Natural-healing enthusiasts and vinegar fans continue to honor and use many of those folk remedies. Vinegar's potential for treating or preventing major medical problems is of interest to almost everyone. But apple cider vinegar in particular has also has been cherished as a home remedy for some common minor ailments for centuries. In this chapter, we'll look at some of those conditions and suggested remedies. Although they're not life-or-death issues, these minor health problems can be uncomfortable, and there is often little modern medicine can offer in the way of a cure. So you may want to give apple cider vinegar a shot to determine for yourself if it can help. (It's always best when trying any remedy for the first time to run it past your doctor to be sure there is no reason you should not try it.)

CAUTIONS

Vinegar is acidic. As you will notice, most home remedies call for dilution of vinegar with water before it is placed on the skin. Do not leave vinegar or vinegar solutions on your skin for long periods of time; rinse them off with water.

Some home remedies combine apple cider vinegar with honey. Do not give these or any other honey-containing food or beverage to children younger than two years of age. Honey can carry a bacterium that can cause a kind of food poisoning called infant botulism and may also cause allergic reactions in very young children.

ACHES AND SORE MUSCLES

You've made your New Year's resolution: You are going to get in shape. Never mind that the last time you exercised was at a charity walk a few years ago and that the very expensive treadmill you bought is now buried underneath a pile of laundry. Twenty pounds and three kids ago you were an aerobics queen, so you know what it's like to feel, and look, better. So you venture into your local health club and decide to try the low/high aerobics class for people who have been out of circulation for a while. You think you can keep up with the twenty-something girls, so you grapevine and kick and half-jack with the beat for 50 minutes. By the time you get home, though, your muscles have gone on strike. The next day you can barely muster enough strength to make it out of bed, and you spend the day walking like you've been riding the range a bit too long. You'll take it slower next time. But what can you do right now to ease the pain? Consider turning to apple cider vinegar!

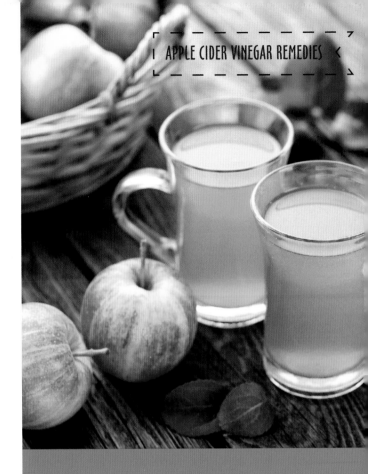

One general tonic for remaining healthy and alert well into the golden years combines good nutrition with vinegar. Maintain a well-balanced diet, and drink a glass of water mixed with 1 teaspoon honey and 1 teaspoon apple cider vinegar at each of your 3 meals a day.

MUSCLE MAYHEM

The vast array of muscles in your body is what allows you to do something as simple as picking up a fork or as complicated as a kickboxing routine. Muscles are a complex weave of fibers that work with your brain and skeletal system to give you the agility to return that volley across the tennis court. When you're taking care to stretch and strengthen your muscles, they are your greatest ally. But when they don't work like they should or they get injured, you end up with a very painful problem on your hands.

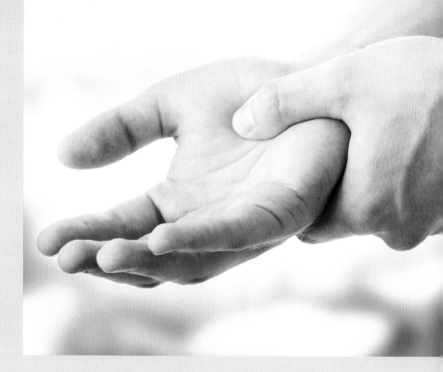

Strains are one of the most common reasons for aching muscles. When you strain a muscle, it means you've worked it too hard, causing the muscle fibers to pull and tear. If you haven't worked out for a while and then head back full throttle without preparing your muscles for the trauma they're about to experience, or if you're an experienced exerciser and you don't warm up properly, you risk getting a strained muscle. At best, a strained muscle will leave you sore for a few days; at worst, you could end up with a "pulled" muscle, one whose fibers have been totally torn. Another common muscle malady is cramps, or spasms. Muscle cramps happen when the muscle isn't getting enough blood, and in response to the restricted blood flow the muscle shortens and tightens. The slowdown in blood flow can be caused by a variety of problems:

- A deficiency in essential nutrients for maximum muscle power, such as sodium, calcium, and potassium
- Depletion of the muscles' energy supply of glycogen
- Overworked muscles
- Holding the same position for too long

Whatever the reason, when blood doesn't reach your muscles the way it should, your muscles can turn into balls of pain. Your first priority is to give your muscles some rest. But you also want to seek some relief!

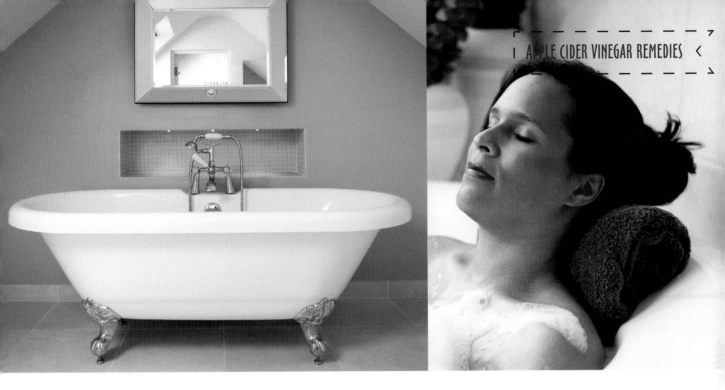

REMEDIES

Add 1 cup apple cider vinegar to a bathtub of warm water. Soak in tub for at least 15 minutes.

Boil 1 cup apple cider vinegar and add 1 teaspoon ground red pepper during boil. Cool this mixture, then apply it in a compress to sore area. Make sure pepper doesn't irritate the skin. The compress should make the area feel warm but not burning.

Try this liniment during a rubdown to relieve achy muscles and arthritis pain: Mix 1 cup apple cider vinegar, 1 cup extra virgin olive oil, and 2 egg whites. Massage into the painful parts; use a clean cotton cloth to wipe off any excess.

In folk medicine some herbs have been labeled "counterirritants." These herbs stimulate blood flow to the skin and the muscles underneath. One common counterirritant in folk healing is mustard seeds. Try this mustard plaster when your muscles ache.

- Crush the seeds of white or brown mustard.
- Moisten with vinegar and sprinkle with flour.
- Spread mixture on a cloth, and cover with a second cloth.
- Lay the moist side on the painful area, and leave on for 20 minutes.
(Remove the plaster if it becomes painful.)

ATHLETE'S FOOT

Athlete's foot itches, burns, and is downright ugly to look at. But it's not a condition unique to athletes. Blame the misnomer on the ad man who gave it its name in the 1930s. In fact, athlete's foot, or *tinea pedis,* is the most common fungal infection of the skin. This fungus loves moist places, especially the soft, warm, damp skin between the toes. Certainly the athlete's locker room environment, with its steamy showers, is a good place for the fungus to thrive. But *tinea pedis* is actually present on most people's skin all the time, just waiting for the right opportunity to develop into an infection.

So what causes athlete's foot to rear its ugly little fungal head? Skin that's irritated, weakened, or continuously moist is primed for an athlete's foot infection. And certain medications, including antibiotics, corticosteroids, birth control pills, and drugs that suppress immune function, can make you more susceptible. People who are obese and those who have diabetes mellitus or a weakened immune system, such as those with AIDS, also are at increased risk. And some people may be genetically pre-disposed to developing athlete's foot.

Anyone can get athlete's foot—and most people will at some time in their lives. Teenage and adult males, though, are the most susceptible. People who spend a lot of time barefoot, women, and children under the age of 12 have the lowest risk.

SIGNS AND SYMPTOMS

Just because you're not in the high risk category doesn't mean you're safe. Here's how you can tell whether you have an athlete's foot infection:

• Itching, scaling, red skin

• Red, cracking, peeling skin between the toes

• Dry, flaking skin

• Blisters

• Unpleasant and unusual foot odor

KEEP IT FROM SPREADING

In extreme cases, the fungus that causes athlete's foot can spread to other moist areas of the body, such as the groin and even the armpits. So take precautions when coming into contact with that athlete's foot. Be sure to wash your hands with soap and water after contact. Keep your linens and towels clean, and never wear the same pair of socks twice without first washing them. You can also spread athlete's foot with contaminated sheets, towels, and clothing.

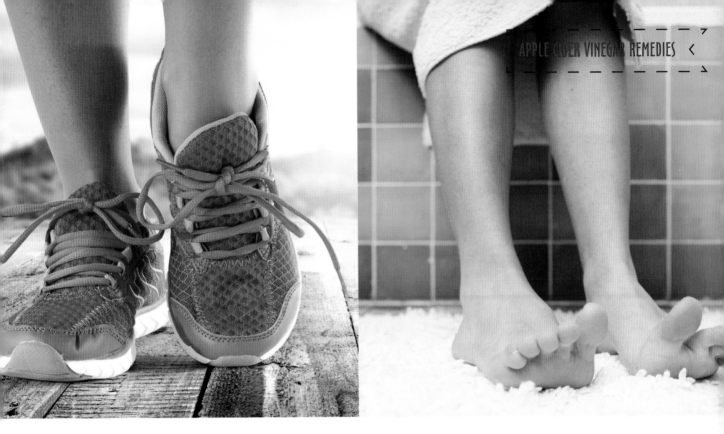

REMEDIES

Mix equal parts apple cider (or regular) vinegar and ethyl alcohol. Dab on the affected areas.

Create an environment that is inhospitable to the fungus that causes the condition. The Amish traditionally use a footbath of vinegar and water to discourage the growth of athlete's foot fungus. To try this remedy, mix one cup of vinegar into two quarts of water in a basin or pan. Soak your feet in this solution every night for 15 to 30 minutes, using a fresh solution each night. Or, if you prefer, mix up a solution using one cup of vinegar and one cup of water. Apply the solution to the affected parts of your feet with a cotton ball. Let your feet dry completely before putting on socks and/or shoes.

For other remedies using essential oils, see page 91 and 96.

BITES AND STINGS

With billions of bugs out there, you're bound to get bit or stung sometime in your life. Typically, the worst reactions are to bees, yellow jackets, hornets, wasps, and fire ants. Other nasty creatures, such as blackflies, horseflies, black or red (not fire) ants, and mosquitoes, also bite and sting, but their venom usually does not cause as intense a reaction. No matter who attacks, once you're zapped the body reacts with redness, itching, pain, and swelling at the bite site. These symptoms may last for a few minutes or a few hours. Thankfully, relief is as close as the kitchen.

Warning! The remedies apply to bites and stings from the insects listed above. A health provider should treat those from snakes, spiders, scorpions, ticks, centipedes, and animals. If the person bitten has a known allergy to insect venom or begins to exhibit signs of a serious allergic reaction, such as widespread hives, swelling of the face or mouth, difficulty breathing, or loss of consciousness, skip the home remedies and seek immediate medical attention.

REMEDIES

No matter whether it's the white or the apple cider variety, vinegar turns insect sting pain into a thing of the past. Mix one tablespoon each of vinegar and baking soda. Apply the paste, and leave it on the sting as long as possible. Apply more, if necessary.

You can also use vinegar mixed with cornstarch to make a paste. Apply paste to a bee sting or bug bite and let dry.

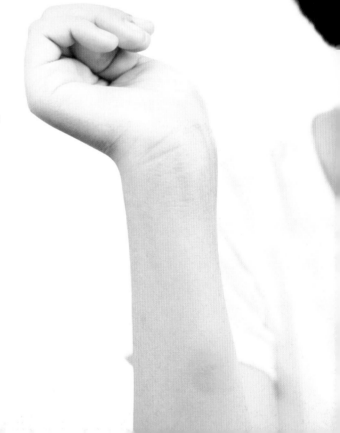

BRONCHITIS

That nasty cold has been hanging on much longer than it should, and day by day it seems to be getting worse. Your chest hurts, you gurgle when you breathe, and you're coughing so much yellow, green, or gray mucus that your throat is raw. These symptoms are letting you know that your cold has probably turned into a respiratory infection called bronchitis, an inflammation of the little branches and tubes of your windpipe that also makes them swell. No wonder breathing has become such a chore. Your air passages are too puffy to carry air very easily.

Acute bronchitis can include these other symptoms, too:

• Wheezing

• Shortness of breath

• Fever or chills

• General aches and pains

• Upper chest pain

Bronchitis is not contagious since it's a secondary infection that develops when your immune system is weakened by a cold or the flu. Some people are prone to developing it, some are not. Those at the top of the risk list have respiratory problems already, such as asthma, allergies, and emphysema. People who have a weakened immune system also are more prone to bronchitis. But anyone can develop it, and most people do at one time or another.

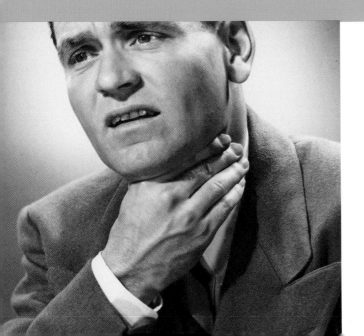

REMEDY

The xanthine derivatives in coffee are good bronchodilators. To cut down on mucus problems, add 1 teaspoon apple cider vinegar and 2 drops peppermint oil to a cup of black coffee, either instant or brewed. Drink 1 cup in the morning and evening.

27

COLDS

E very year Americans will suffer through more than one billion colds. That's one billion runny noses, coughs, sneezes, aches, and sore throats. Colds make such frequent appearances that the infection has come to be known as the "common cold."

Small children are the most likely to catch a cold: Most kids will have six to ten colds a year. That's because their young immune systems combined with the germy confines of school and day-care situations make them prime targets for the virus. The upside of having so many colds as a child is that you develop immunities to some of the 200 viruses that cause colds. As a result, adults get an average of only two to four colds a year. By the time most people reach age 60, they're down to about one cold per year. Women, however, especially women between 20 and 30 years old, get more colds than men.

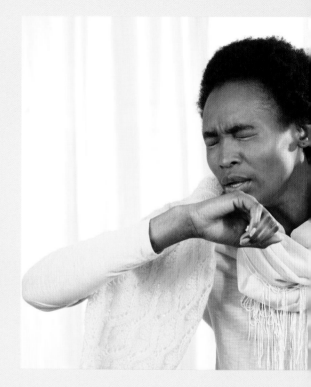

HOW DO COLDS BEAT A PATH TO YOUR DOOR?

Viruses are like the bully that torments all the kids on the playground. After entering the mucous layer of your nose and throat, the cold virus strong-arms your cells until they let the virus take over, forcing the cells to produce thousands of new virus particles. But the virus is not the reason your throat begins throbbing and your nose starts flowing like Niagara Falls. Your immune system is responsible for that. As the virus begins replicating, the body gets the message that it's time to go into battle.

The little soldiers of the body, the white blood cells, run to the body's rescue. One of the weapons the white blood cells use in their virus war are immune system chemicals called kinins. During the battle the kinins tell the body to go into defensive mode. So that runny nose is really your body fighting back against the cursed virus. That should make you feel a little better while you lie on the couch surrounded by tissues.

Because there are so many viruses that cause colds, the exact virus that you contracted is not easily pinned down. The most likely culprit in most colds is a rhinovirus (rhino is a Greek word meaning "nose"). There are over 110 specific rhinoviruses, and they are behind 30 to 35 percent of most colds.

The second most common reason for that aching head is a coronavirus. These are especially common in adults. An unknown viral assailant causes 30 to 50 percent of colds, and about 10 to 15 percent of colds are caused by a virus that will probably lead to something more serious, such as the flu.

HOW COLDS ARE SPREAD

The cold virus can take many routes to its ultimate destination—your cells. Most people are contagious a day before and two to four days after their symptoms start. There are typically three ways a cold virus is spread:

- Touching someone who has the virus on them. The virus can live for three hours on skin.
- Touching something that contains the virus. Cold viruses can live three hours on objects.
- Inhaling the virus through airborne transmission. It may sound implausible, but if someone sitting next to you sneezes while you are inhaling, voilà! It's likely you'll get a cold.

One study found that kids tend to get colds from more direct contact while adults tend to get colds from airborne viruses (moms of young children can expect to get colds both ways).

Research has also found that emotional stress, allergies that affect the nasal passages or throat, and menstrual cycles may make you more susceptible to catching a cold.

Apple cider vinegar can't be used to cure your cold, alas, but it has been used traditionally to help alleviate troublesome symptoms.

REMEDIES

For a sore throat, mix one teaspoon of apple cider vinegar into a glass of water; gargle with a mouthful of the solution and then swallow it, repeating until you've finished all the solution in the glass.

For a natural cough syrup, mix half a tablespoon apple cider vinegar with half a tablespoon honey and swallow. Or mix ¼ cup honey and apple cider vinegar; pour into a jar or bottle that can be tightly sealed. Shake well before each use. Take 1 tablespoon every 4 hours. If cough persists for more than a week, see a physician. (Do not give it or any other honey-containing food or beverage to children younger than two years of age. Honey can carry a bacterium that can cause a kind of food poisoning called infant botulism and may also cause allergic reactions in very young children.)

You can add a quarter-cup of apple cider vinegar to the recommended amount of water in your room vaporizer to help with congestion.

To alleviate a sore throat and also thin mucus, gargle with apple cider vinegar that has a little salt and ground black pepper added to it.

Inhaling the fumes of vinegar is a cold remedy as old as ancient Greece. The famous physician Hippocrates recommended the treatment for coughs and respiratory infections. In a jar, pour half a cup of boiling water over half a cup of vinegar. Gently inhale the steam, being careful not to burn yourself.

Mix 1 tablespoon of honey and 1 tablespoon of apple cider vinegar with 8 ounces of hot water. Use as often as desired.

CONSTIPATION

Nothing's moving, even though you know you have to move your bowels. Everything in your body is sending you that signal. You feel bloated and uncomfortable pressure, but when you try to go, nothing happens. Or, if you do finally go, it hurts.

Constipation occurs for many different reasons. Stress, lack of exercise, certain medications, artificial sweeteners, and a diet that's lacking fiber or fluids can each be the culprit. Certain medical conditions such as an underactive thyroid, irritable bowel syndrome, diabetes, and cancer also can cause constipation. Even age is a factor. The older we get, the more prone we are to the problem.

And constipation is a problem, although it's not an illness. It's simply what happens when bowel movements are delayed, compacted, and difficult to pass.

WHAT'S NORMAL?

Some people mistakenly believe they must have a certain number of bowel movements a day or a week or else they are constipated. That couldn't be further from the truth, although it's a common misconception. What constitutes "normal" is individual and can vary from three bowel movements a day to three a week. You'll know if you're constipated because you'll be straining a lot in the bathroom, you'll produce unusually hard stools, and you'll feel gassy and bloated.

REMEDIES

It's not a good idea to use laxatives as the first line of attack when you're constipated. They can become habit-forming to the point that they damage your colon. Some laxatives inhibit the effectiveness of medications you're already taking, and there are laxatives that cause inflammation to the lining of the intestine. Conventional thinking on laxatives is that if you must take one, find one that's psyllium- or fiber-based. Psyllium is a natural fiber that's much more gentle on the system than ingredients in many of the other products available today. Or, simply look to apple cider vinegar for relief.

Mix 1 teaspoon apple cider vinegar and 1 teaspoon honey in a glass of water and drink.

Safflower, soybean, or other vegetable oil can be just the cure you need, as they have a lubricating action in the intestines. Take 2 to 3 tablespoons a day until the problem is gone. If you don't like taking it straight, mix the oil with herbs and vinegar to use as salad dressing. The combination of the oil and the fiber from the salad ought to fix you right up.

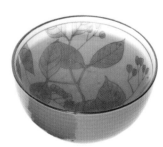

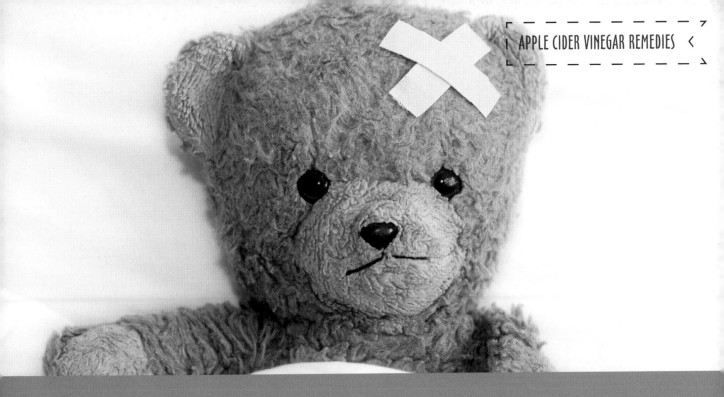

CUTS AND SCRAPES

You're hurrying along and the front of your shoe catches on a crack in the cement, sending you tumbling to the ground. When you get up, you find that not only is your ego bruised, but you've managed to peel away the skin on your elbows and knees. You've got yourself a collection of painful scrapes.

You scramble home to prepare the appetizer tray for the guests who will be arriving any minute. You have just one more carrot to slice when, "Ouch!"—your knife slips and slices not the carrot, but your finger. You've got a cut.

An amazing number of things happen when you cut or scrape yourself. When you disrupt the skin, a clear, antibody-containing fluid from the blood, called serum, leaks into the wound. The area around the cut or scrape becomes red, indicating that more blood is moving into the wound site, bringing with it nutrients and infection-fighting white blood cells. Nearby lymph nodes may swell. After a few days, pus (which contains dead white blood cells, dead bacteria, and other debris from the body's inflammatory response to infection) may form. And finally, a scab develops to protect the injury while it heals.

Even being extra careful, you can't always avoid the scrapes and cuts of life. But you can learn how to care for them and speed their healing.

STEPS TO TAKE

Stop the bleeding. When you get a cut or scrape, the first thing to do (after admonishing yourself for being so clumsy) is to stop the bleeding. Use a clean cloth or tissue to apply pressure to the wound. If possible, elevate the wound above the heart to slow the blood flow. Don't use a tourniquet.

Wash up. One of the most important things you can do in treating a cut or scrape is to make sure you cleanse it thoroughly with soap and water.

Bring on the antibacterial ointment. Polysporin, Neosporin, and Bactine are examples of anti-bacterial ointments available without a prescription.

Close and cover. Properly closing the skin is important in cuts that are an eighth to a quarter inch wide in order to make the cut heal faster and to reduce the chances of scarring. Be sure that you have thoroughly cleansed the cut before attempting to close it. Line up the edges of the cut, then apply butterfly strips or an adhesive bandage to keep the cut closed. Keeping the cut or scrape covered will reduce the change of infection or further injury.

You want the bandage or covering to be tight enough to protect, but not so tight that it seals out all air and causes the wound to become too moist.

Keep it clean. Remove the bandage every day and wash the wound with soap and water. Then re-cover it with a clean bandage.

Don't let it dry out. One of the myths about cuts and scrapes is that a thick, crusty scab is good. Not so. The wound should stay moist. If a scab forms, don't pick at it; this disrupts the skin and can introduce bacteria. Instead, soak off crusty scabs with a solution of one tablespoon of white vinegar to one pint of water. The mildly acidic solution is soothing and helps kill bacteria.

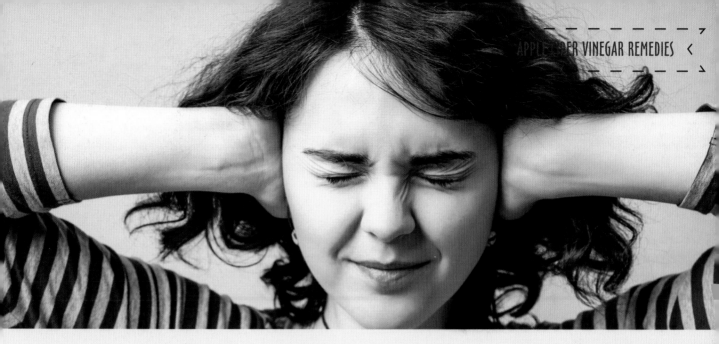

HEADACHE

The day starts with screaming kids, continues slowly onward with stop 'n' go traffic, and ends on a sour note with an angry boss. By this point, you are ready to chop your head off in order to relieve the pounding pain.

You can take a little comfort in knowing that almost everyone has had such a day...and such a headache. Yet some people fare worse than others do. An estimated 45 million Americans get chronic, recurring headaches, while as many as 18 million of those suffer from painful, debilitating migraines.

THREE KINDS OF HEADACHES

Although there are nearly two dozen types of headaches, they all fall into three basic categories: tension, vascular, and organic.

Tension headaches, the most common of the trio, cause a dull, nonthrobbing pain, usually accompanied by tightness in the scalp or neck. Triggers range from depression to everyday stresses such as screaming kids and traffic jams.

Vascular headaches are more intense, severe, throbbing, and piercing: They take first prize for pain. Cluster and migraine headaches fall into this category. Triggers for cluster headaches are unknown, although excessive smoking and alcohol consumption can ignite them. Migraines are thought to be caused by heredity, diet, stress, menstruation, and environmental factors such as cigarette smoke.

Less common are organic headaches, in which pain becomes increasingly worse and is accompanied by other symptoms, such as vomiting, coordination problems, visual disturbances, or speech or personality changes. Triggers include tumors, infections, or diseases of the brain, eyes, ears, and nose. If you are prone to the usual tension headache, head to the kitchen for a variety of remedies that can help your throbbing head.

33

REMEDIES

Ease a headache by lying down and applying a compress dipped in a mixture of half warm water and half apple cider vinegar to the temples.

Use above treatment for treating a headache, but try an herbal vinegar such as lavender to provide aromatic relief.

If you suffer from recurring headaches, you might want to plant a little feverfew in your herb garden (or grow the herb in a windowsill pot). This lovely, easy-to-nurture herb has long been used as a headache remedy, especially for migraines. Feverfew causes blood vessels to dilate and inhibits the secretion of substances that cause pain and inflammation (such as histamine and serotonin) through the substance parthenolide. You have two choices when it comes to taking feverfew: eating it raw or drinking it in tea. If you do prefer the au naturel way, add 2 to 3 of the leaves to a salad dressed with vinegar.

FEVER

Fever is a good thing. It's your body's attempt to kill off invading bacteria and other nasty organisms that can't survive the heat. The hypothalamus, which is the body's thermostat, senses the assault on the body and turns up the heat much the way you turn up the thermostat when you feel cold. It's a simple defense mechanism, and the sweat that comes with a fever is merely a way to cool the body down.

It used to be standard medical practice to knock that fever out as quickly as possible. Not so anymore. The value of fever is recognized, and since a fever will

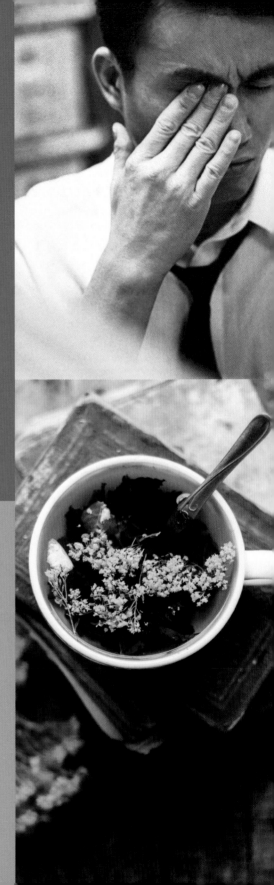

34

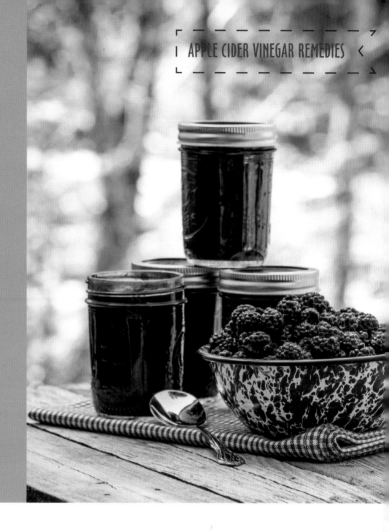

usually subside when the infection that's causing it runs its course, modern thinking is to ride out that fever, especially if it stays under 102°F in adults. However, if a fever is making you uncomfortable or interfering with your ability to eat, drink, or sleep, treat it. Your body needs adequate nutrition, hydration, and rest to fight the underlying cause of the fever.

Fever is a symptom, not an illness, and so there's no specific cure. But there is one traditional remedy involving vinegar that may help you feel better.

REMEDY

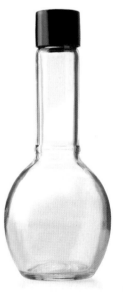

Blackberry vinegar is a great fever elixir, but it takes several days to prepare. Pour cider vinegar over a pound or two of blackberries, then cover the container and store it in a cool, dark place for three days. Strain for a day, since it takes time for all the liquid to drain from the berries, and collect the liquid in another container. Then add 2 cups sugar to each 2 ½ cups juice. Bring to a boil, then simmer for 5 minutes while you skim the scum off the top. Cool and store in an airtight jar in a cool place. Mix 1 teaspoonful with water to quench the thirst caused by a fever.

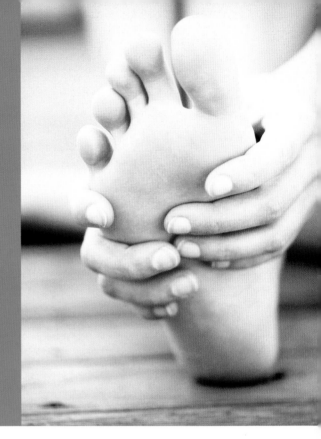

FOOT CARE

Overworked and taken for granted; that's the lot of the lowly foot. But feet are a marvelous work of nature and an absolute architectural wonder. Each one of your feet is made up of 26 bones, 33 joints, 107 ligaments, and 31 tendons. Together, they comprise one-quarter of all the bones in your body.

Every day, on average, we take about 10,000 steps. That adds up to four hikes around the planet during a lifetime. And each time a step is taken, the impact of hitting the ground is about four times your body weight. No wonder, then, that 70 percent of us experience foot and ankle problems at some time. Here are some remedies for common foot problems.

REMEDIES

For tough toenails, soak your feet in equal parts vinegar and water to soften and clean the nail before you clip.

Swollen feet can be annoying when your favorite shoes don't fit. Here's an easy fix to reduce the swelling, which is a buildup of fluid in the tissues called edema. Mix 4 teaspoons cider vinegar in a large glass of water. Drink three times a day. (Warning: If you are taking a diuretic medication, consult your doctor before trying this remedy.)

To soothe tendinitis, sprains, strains, and general foot aches, alternate hot and cold vinegar wraps. First, heat equal amounts of vinegar and water. Soak a towel in the mixture, wring it out, and wrap it around your foot. Leave it wrapped for five minutes. Then mix equal parts vinegar and cold water and follow the same procedure. Repeat this entire sequence three times.

For sprains or sore feet, take a handful of sage leaves and rub them in your palm. (This is called bruising, and it releases the herb's curative chemicals.) Put them in a saucepan with $2/3$ cup cider vinegar. Boil, then simmer for five minutes. After removing from the heat, soak a cloth in the solution and apply it to a sprain or sore foot, as hot as tolerable.

For foot odor, soak your feet several times a week in an apple cider or plain vinegar bath. Mix $1/3$ cup vinegar into a bowl of warm water. Soak for 10 to 15 minutes.

HEARTBURN

Boy, oh boy, did you do it this time. You added that heaping second helping to all the platter pickings you couldn't resist, and what do you have? Indigestion (an incomplete or imperfect digestion), that's what. And it may be accompanied by pain, nausea, vomiting, heartburn, gas, and belching. All this because you couldn't resist temptation. But don't worry. It happens to everybody, and it goes away.

So, now that you've eaten until you're about ready to burst, what's next? The couch, maybe? Stretch out, let your digestive system do its thing, take a nap?

Wrong! The worst thing you can do after a binge is to lie down. That can cause heartburn, also known as acid indigestion. Whatever you call it, it's the feeling you get when digestive acid escapes your stomach and irritates the esophagus, the tube that leads from your throat to your stomach. After you eat, heartburn can also fire up when you:

• Bend forward
• Exercise
• Strain muscles

WHY ACID BACKS UP

Occasionally the acid keeps on coming until you have a mouthful of something bitter and acidy. You may have some pain in your gut, too, or in your chest. Along with that acid may come a belch, one that may bring even more of that stomach acid with it.

The purpose of stomach acid is to break down the foods we eat so our body can digest them. Our stomachs have a protective lining that shields it from those acids, but the esophagus does not have that protection. Normally that's not a problem, because after we swallow food, it passes down the esophagus, through a sphincter, and into the stomach. The sphincter then closes.

Occasionally, though, the muscles of that sphincter are weakened and it doesn't close properly or it doesn't close all the way. Scarring from an ulcer or frequent episodes of acid reflux (when the acid comes back up), stomach pressure from overeating, obesity, and pregnancy can all cause this glitch in the lower esophageal sphincter (LES). And when the LES gets a glitch and allows the gastric acid to splash out of the stomach, you get heartburn.

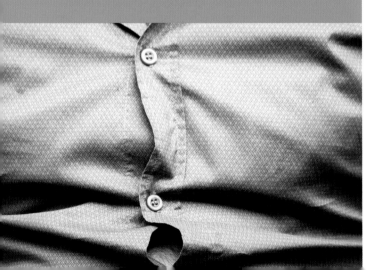

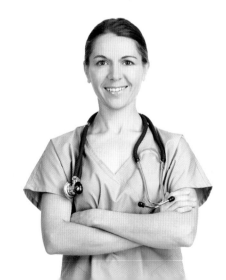

Generally, heartburn isn't serious. In fact, small amounts of reflux are normal and most people don't even notice it because the swallowing we do causes saliva to wash the acids right back down into the stomach where they belong. When the stomach starts shooting back amounts that are larger than normal, especially on a regular basis or over a prolonged period of time, that's when the real trouble begins, and simple heartburn can turn into esophageal inflammation or bleeding.

Who's prone to heartburn? Just about anybody. According to the National Digestive Diseases Clearinghouse, 25 million adults suffer from heartburn daily and about 60 million Americans get gastroesophageal reflux and heartburn at least once a month.

REMEDY

There are several prescription medicines available for the treatment of long-term or serious heartburn or acid reflux, and over-the-counter remedies are available at your pharmacy, too. But you can also try this home remedy.

Mix 1 tablespoon apple cider vinegar, 1 tablespoon honey, and 1 cup warm water. Drink at the first sign of heartburn.

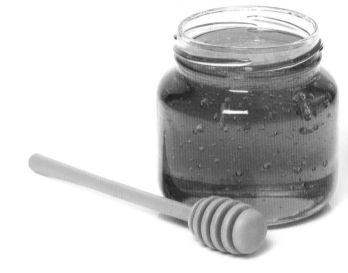

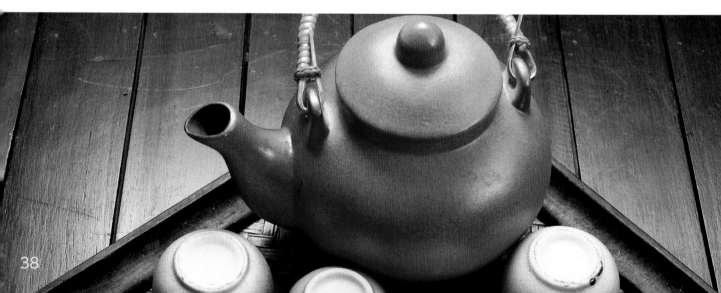

ITCHES

To scratch or not to scratch, that is the question. When confronted with an itch, most of us tend to throw self-discipline out the door and scratch to our skin's content. While that may prove momentarily satisfying, scratching excessively can injure your skin. And if you break the skin, you leave yourself open to infection. Itching, medically known as pruritus, is caused by stimuli bugging some part of our skin. There are a lot of places to bother on the body, too. The average adult has 20 square feet (2 square meters) of skin, all open to the world of irritants. When something bothers our skin, an itch is a built-in defense mechanism that alerts the body that someone is knocking. We respond to an itch with a scratch, as most people want to remove the problem. But the scratching can also set you up for the "itch-scratch" cycle, where one leads to the other endlessly.

An itch can range from a mild nuisance to a disrupting, damaging, and sleep-depriving fiasco. Itches happen for many reasons, including allergic reactions; sunburns; insect bites; poison ivy; reactions to chemicals, soaps, and detergents; medication; dry weather; skin infections; and even aging. More serious itches, such as those caused by psoriasis or other diseases, are not covered here. Fortunately, scratching isn't the only solution to an itch.

REMEDIES

To relieve itchy skin, add 1 cup apple cider vinegar to a bathtub of warm water. Soak in tub for at least 15 minutes.

Use your freezer to soothe and cool just about any kind of skin itchiness, be it from sunburn, a bug bite, or a rash. Fill each compartment of an empty, clean foam egg carton with apple cider vinegar; freeze. When the itch gets insane, pop out a vinegar cube and rub it over the spot.

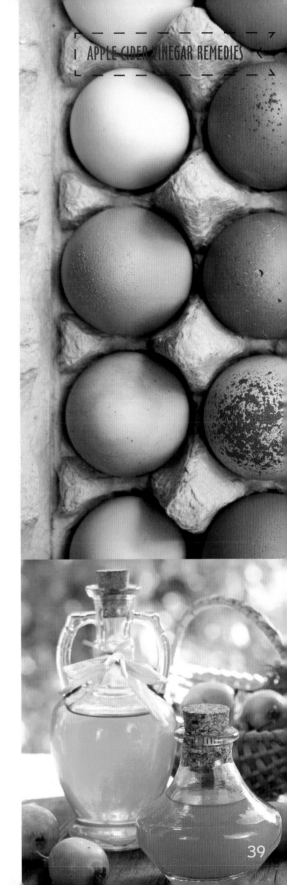

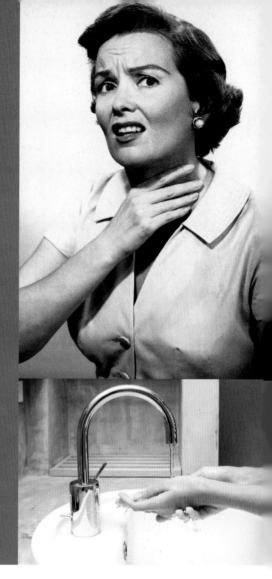

LARYNGITIS

Have you been verbally abusing your voice? Too much vocal enthu-siasm at a sports event can set you up for swollen vocal cords and no voice the next day. But that's not the only way to cause laryngitis—the result of inflammation of the voice box and voice folds. More often, laryngitis is caused by an upper respiratory infection, usually viral, such as the common cold. Surprisingly, some cases of laryngitis are caused by heartburn, especially in the elderly. During the night, the acid-rich contents of the stomach come back up the throat and cause irritation.

SOUNDS AND SYMPTOMS

When we speak, two membranes, known as the vocal cords, vibrate to produce sounds. Hoarseness, the main sign of laryngitis, is an indicator that something with the vocal chords is wrong, swollen, irritated, or in-fected. Besides hoarseness, symptoms of acute, or short-term, laryngi-tis also include a painful or scratchy feeling in the throat, a loss of range in the voice, and fatigue. You may also have the annoying feeling that you must constantly clear your throat. In heartburn-induced laryngitis, symptoms include waking up with a bad taste in the mouth, feeling like something is sticking in the throat, constant throat clearing, and hoarse-ness that gradually improves during the day.

REMEDIES

Viruses and bacteria dread an acidic environment, so why not make your mouth one big, albeit weak, acid bath? Gargling with vinegar, a weak acid, can help wipe out many infectious organisms. Pour equal amounts of vinegar and water into a cup, mix, and gargle two to four times a day. You can also gargle with straight vinegar, but some people find it too strong, especially at first

Laryngitis can be caused by a viral infection and is easily spread by hand-to-hand contact or by touching contaminated surfaces. Avoiding such germs is one of the best ways to prevent laryngitis. If you or someone around you has a cold, be extra vigilant about washing your hands with warm water and soap. Clean common surfaces, such as the telephone and door handles, with vinegar and a clean cloth.

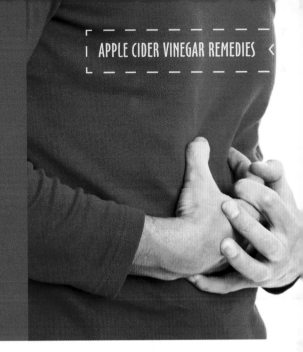

STOMACH UPSET

You and the spouse celebrated your promotion with dinner at your favorite barbecue joint. You've been working hard for months, you think, so you deserve to cut loose a little. On the way home you groan and mutter that you wish you had stopped after that first barbecue platter. Your wife shrugs her shoulders. You both know the price for your revelry will be a painful night of bloating, gas, and heartburn.

But sometimes your tummy can turn on you even when you haven't been making one too many trips to the buffet table. It's important to know what's normal tummy trouble and what's something to take more seriously.

THE DIGESTIVE DANCE

When you eat something, the digestive process begins right away in your mouth. Your salivary glands produce digestive juices that lubricate your food and prepare fat for digestion. The food travels through your esophagus into your stomach, where digestive juices continue to break food down even further so it can travel on to the small intestine. The pancreas and liver secrete other digestive juices that flow into the small intestines. In the small intestine, vital nutrients including vitamins, minerals, water, salt, carbohydrates, and proteins are sucked out of the food and absorbed into your body. By the time your dinner makes its way to the large intestines, it's mostly bulk and water. The large intestines absorb the water and help you get rid of the, umm, excess.

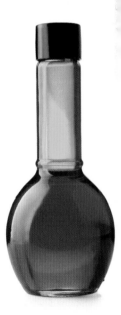

But sometimes things in the digestive system go awry and cause indigestion, a catchall term that means you simply have trouble digesting your food. When you eat too much, or you eat the wrong foods, you may get one of a number of indigestion symptoms mentioned above: nausea, vomiting, heartburn, bloating, or gas. Those unpleasant feelings may send you running to the drugstore for relief, and if they do, you've got plenty of company. The American Gastroenterological Association says that digestive problems are one of the most common reasons Americans take over-the-counter medications. Indigestion can be a symptom of something more serious, such as gastritis, an ulcer, severe heartburn, irritable bowel syndrome, or diverticulitis. But if it's just the result of overdoing it at dinner, apple cider vinegar may be able to help.

41

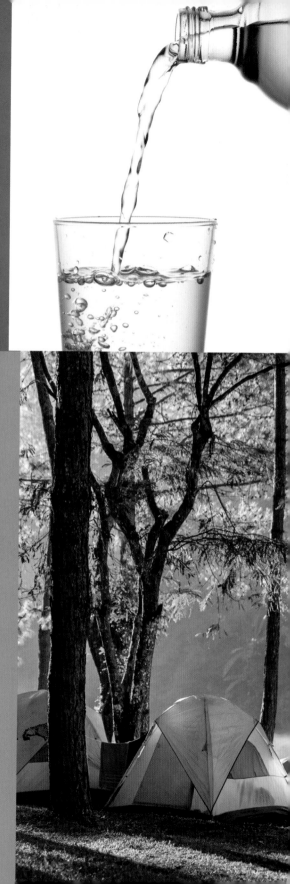

REMEDY

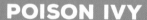

To settle minor stomach upset, try a simple cider vinegar tonic with a meal. Drinking a mixture of a spoonful of vinegar in a glass of water is said to improve digestion and ease minor stomach upset by stimulating digestive juices.

POISON IVY

Contact with poison ivy, poison oak, or poison sumac often goes hand-in-hand with camping and other outdoor activities. Outdoor enthusiasts by the tentful have had to cut trips short after an unfortunate encounter with one of this threesome. The problem stems from the plant's colorless oil called urushiol. Whenever one of these plants is cut, crushed, stepped on, sat on, grabbed, rolled on, kicked, or disturbed, the oil is released. Once on the victim, the toxic oil penetrates the skin and a rash appears within 12 to 48 hours after exposure. This is a true allergic reaction to compounds in the urushiol. The rash starts as small bumps and progresses into enlarged, itchy blisters. No body part is immune to the oil, although areas most often irritated are the face, arms, hands, legs, and genitals.

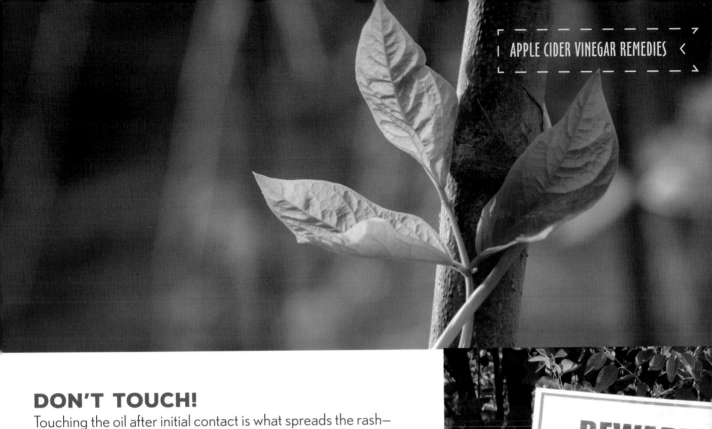

DON'T TOUCH!

Touching the oil after initial contact is what spreads the rash—something easily done. For example, pretend you unknowingly walk over poison ivy and the oily residue sticks like glue to your hiking boot. Later, you remove the boot, unwittingly touching the residue in the process. Since few people wash their hands after removing boots, the oil easily spreads from the hands, to the face, and even to the genital area should you make the unfortunate decision to use the bathroom. The damage is done by the time the rash breaks out. Touching the rash once it appears does not spread the oil—or the rash.

WARNING! Since poison plant oils don't just disappear, it's crucial to wash anything that has had contact with the victim or the oil, including clothing, boots, pets, other people, sleeping bags, fishing poles, walking sticks, etc. Use gloves when cleaning pets, people, and objects that may have had contact with the oil.

Outdoor expeditions need not be ruined if people learn to recognize the terrible threesome. Here are some pointers.

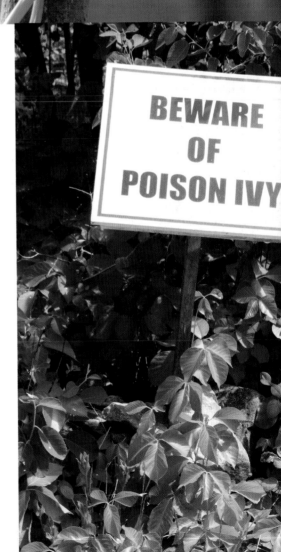

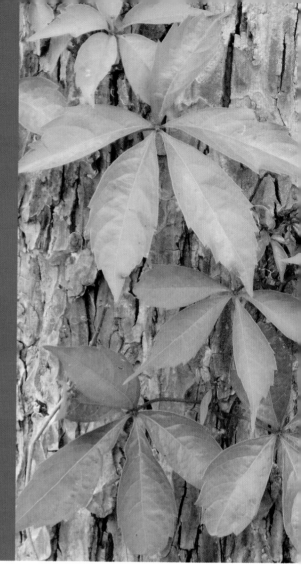

Poison ivy. Poison ivy plants have serrated, pointed leaves that appear in groups of three leaflets. The leaves are green in summer but are reddish in spring and fall. While their appearance can vary, poison ivy plants are found everywhere in the United States. In the East, Midwest, and South, it grows as a climbing vine. In the West and northern states, poison ivy resembles a shrub. Poison ivy rarely appears above 5,000 feet.

Poison oak. Like poison ivy, poison oak has leaves of three and the shrub's size differs depending on location. In the Southeast it appears as a small shrub, while in the West, poison oak appears as a large shrub. It has greenish-white berries and oaklike leaves.

Poison sumac. The leafy one of this threesome is poison sumac, a small shrub with two rows of 7 to 13 leaflets. Sumac prefers swampy bogs of northern states and swamps in southern states. Its leaves are smooth-edged and remain red; the plant has cream-colored berries. Unlike poison ivy and oak, poison sumac does not produce leaves in groups of three.

Even experts can be fooled by the poisonous three, so here's some relief.

REMEDIES

Be it from plant, insect, or allergic reaction, itches of all sorts are tamed by a simple vinegar rinse. First wash the affected area with soap and lukewarm water, then rinse. Apply vinegar with a cotton ball, rub gently, and rinse.

Before going to bed, pour a cup of baking soda into a lukewarm bath and take a soak.

For a more complex remedy involving essential oils, see page 97.

PSORIASIS

Psoriasis is a noncontagious, chronic skin condition that produces round, dry, scaly patches that are covered with white, gray, or silver-white scales. These patches are called plaques.

Although psoriasis is a mysterious condition (doctors aren't exactly sure what causes it or why it can be mild one day and serious the next), it is common. According to information from the National Institutes of Health, between 5.8 million and 7.5 million Americans have the disease. Psoriasis is also tough to treat because what works for one person may not work for another, and treatments that were once effective for an individual often become ineffective, and vice versa.

REMEDY

One solution that some people have found helpful to try is an apple cider vinegar dip. It's a great soak for affected fingernails and toenails; just pour some in a bowl or cup and dip your nails in for a few minutes. Some people have also had success applying it to plaques using cotton balls.

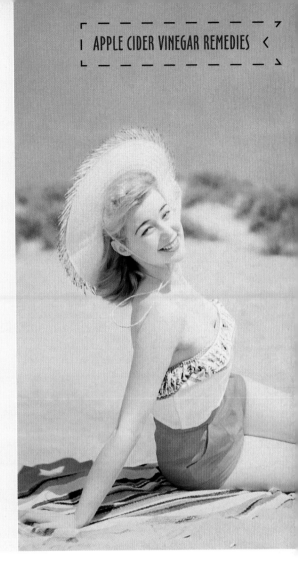

SUNBURN

A sunburn is one of the most common hazards of the great outdoors. The unappealing and painful lobster look results when the amount of exposure to the sun exceeds the ability of the body's protective pigment, melanin, to protect the skin. What makes sunburn different from, say, a household iron burn? The time factor. A sunburn is not immediately apparent. By the time the skin starts to become red, the damage has been done. Pain isn't always instantly noticeable, either.

You may feel glowing after two hours sitting poolside without sun protection. But just wait awhile. You'll change your tune (not to mention color) when the pain sets in, typically 6 to 48 hours after sun exposure. Like household burns, sunburns are summed up by degree. Mild sunburns are deep pink, punctuated by a hot, burning sensation. Moderate sunburns are red, clothing lines are prominent, and the skin itches and stings. Severe sunburns result in bright red skin, blisters, fever, chills, and nausea.

Being burned to a crisp can lead to serious consequences later in life. In fact, one severe, blistering sunburn during childhood doubles your chances of developing malignant melanoma, a deadly form of skin cancer, or other types of skin cancer such as basal cell and squamous cell carcinomas. If cancer doesn't frighten you, then the specter of developing premature wrinkling and age spots just might. Obviously, covering up and applying a waterproof sunscreen with a high SPF (sun protection factor) is the best way to prevent sunburn. But when you slip, you can call on apple cider vinegar for relief.

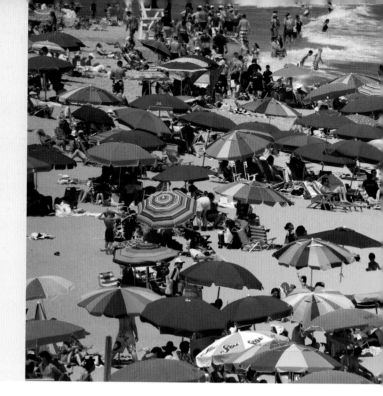

REMEDY

A mixture of white or apple cider vinegar with an equal amount of cool water can be used to bathe a garden-variety sunburn. If no one is around to help you, fill a spray bottle with the solution and spray the affected areas. You can also wear a large, loose-fitting soft cotton T-shirt that has been soaked in the mixture. See another remedy on page 95.

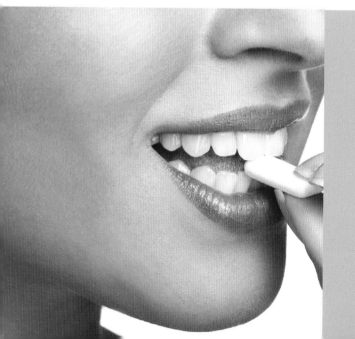

TOOTH CARE

We take those choppers for granted, don't we? Except for that first year or two of life, they've always been there, ready to take on the grueling task of chewing. We douse them with sugar that erodes their enamel, require them to work overtime on foods hard enough to be called petrified, and then we forget the basics our parents taught us: Brush after every meal, and don't eat so many sweets.

Our teeth serve us well when they're in good order, but when something goes wrong, ouch!

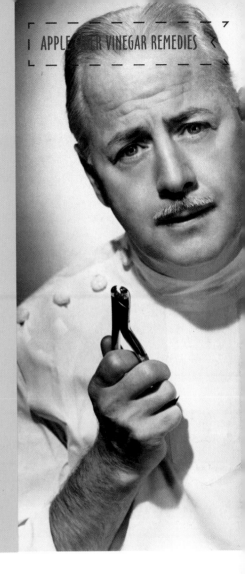

First comes that off-and-on-again little twinge, the one we ignore and hope will disappear. Next comes the sensitivity to hot and cold. And finally the full-out throb that hurts so bad that pulling the tooth out with a piece of string tied to a doorknob doesn't seem like such a bad way out.

Tooth problems hurt like a...toothache, and ultimately the solution comes in a dentist's chair, the drill screaming in your ear, your teeth clenching against the needle being jabbed into your mouth.
Yes, we do abuse our teeth. And what's amazing about that is that overall, we're not neglecting our dental health. On average, 65 percent of all Americans visit their dentist regularly. So what's the deal?

Why the toothache?

• Poor food choices
• Bacteria
• Bad brushing technique
• Not enough flossing
• Heredity
• Lack of professional care

Take your pick, the list is long. But vinegar can help remedy some of your dental dilemmas, from toothache to tooth care.

REMEDIES

Here's an easy but temporary toothache fix. Try rinsing your mouth with a mixture of 4 ounces warm water, 2 tablespoons cider vinegar, and 1 tablespoon salt. If toothache persists, see a dentist.

A refreshing mouthwash can be made with ¼ cup water and ¼ cup apple cider vinegar in a 4-ounce glass. Gargle with this to freshen your mouth and control bad breath.

To brighten dentures, soak them overnight in pure white vinegar.

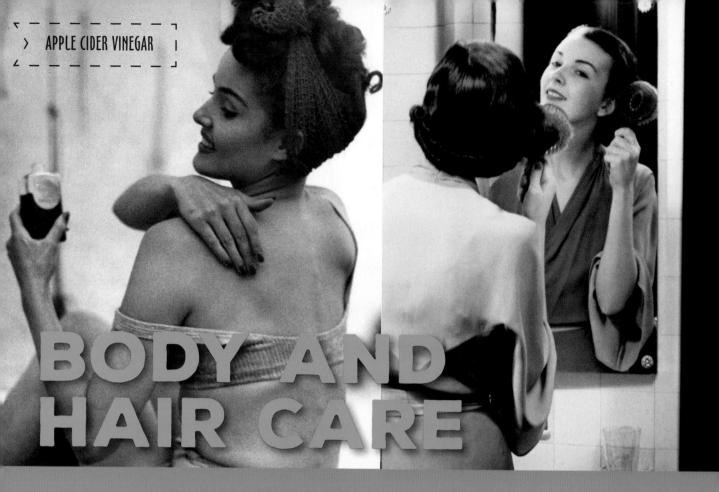

BODY AND HAIR CARE

Apple cider vinegar solutions are wonderful—and inexpensive—additions to your beauty and cleansing regimens. Vinegar can help restore the natural acidity of your skin, which may clear up skin problems. Read on for tips to help you stay relaxed and beautiful without spending a fortune.

CAUTION

Vinegar is acidic. As you will notice, most regimens call for dilution of vinegar with water before it is placed on the skin. Do not leave vinegar or vinegar solutions on your skin for long periods of time; rinse them off with water.

GENERAL SKIN CARE

Make a basic skin toner using a mixture of equal parts apple cider vinegar or distilled white vinegar and water. Keep toner in a small spray bottle and apply after your usual wash.

Vinegar mixed with onion juice may help reduce the appearance of age spots. Mix equal parts of onion juice and vinegar, and dab onto age spots. After several weeks of this routine, spots should lighten.

HERB-SCENTED SKIN TONER

Use 1 part vinegar to 3 parts water, and add the following flower or herb petals of your choice. Spray on skin as desired to freshen.

FOR DRY SKIN:
violet, rose, borage, or jasmine

FOR OILY SKIN:
peppermint, marigold, rosemary, or lavender

FOR SENSITIVE SKIN:
violet, salt burnet, parsley, or borage

FOR NEUTRAL SKIN:
lemon balm, rose, spearmint, or chamomile

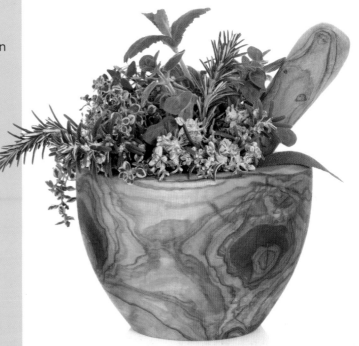

CARING FOR YOUR HANDS

Are your hands a mess from grease, gardening, or generally getting things done? Clean very dirty hands by scrubbing with cornmeal that has been moistened with a little bit of apple cider vinegar. Thoroughly scrub your hands—don't miss a grimy finger, knuckle, nail, or palm. Rinse well and dry; repeat if necessary. Your hands will be soft and smooth—and the dirt will be gone!

Mix equal parts vinegar and hand cream to help chapped hands.

Make your nail polish last longer on your fingers by soaking fingertips for 1 minute in 2 teaspoons vinegar and ½ cup warm water before applying polish.

To remove onion odor from your hands, sprinkle on a little salt, then moisten with a bit of vinegar. Rub hands together, and rinse.

For softer hands, combine 1 gallon white distilled vinegar and herbs and spices like cinnamon, nutmeg, or cardamom. Let mixture sit for 1 month, then strain out spice or herb debris. Pour the fragrant vinegar into an empty, clean bottle with a spray nozzle, or buy a new decorative bottle to keep at your sink. After you wash dishes or when you've had your hands in hot water, spray vinegar mixture on your hands. Regular use of this vinegar spray will soften your hands and make them smell nice, too!

FACIAL CARE

Use a mixture of half apple cider vinegar, half water to clean and tone your face. Then rinse with vinegar diluted with water, and let your face air-dry to seal in moisture.

Control oily skin with a mixture of equal parts apple cider vinegar and cool water. The mixture works as an astringent. You can also freeze this solution into ice cubes and use it as a cooling facial treatment on a hot summer day.

Apple cider vinegar is a great aftershave for men that will keep their skin soft and young looking. Keep a small bottle of it in the medicine cabinet, and splash on your face after shaving.

ASTRINGENT FACIAL SCRUB

$\frac{1}{8}$ cup astringent herbs, such as sage, yarrow, or chamomile, ground fine

$\frac{1}{4}$ cup oatmeal, ground fine, or cornmeal

Cider vinegar

This cleansing preparation is great for oily skin. And you've probably got the ingredients in your kitchen cabinet. Combine herbs and meal, then add enough vinegar to make a paste. Scrub your face with this mixture and rinse with cool water.

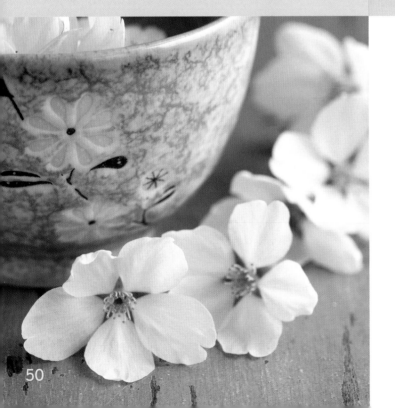

FACIAL TONER FOR OILY COMPLEXIONS

12 drops lemongrass oil

6 drops juniper berry oil

2 drops ylang ylang oil

1 ounce apple cider vinegar

1 ounce aloe vera gel

Combine all of the ingredients in a glass bottle. Give the mixture a good shake and it's done! Apply at least once a day.

FACIAL SPLASHES

Herbal: Boil 1 quart apple cider vinegar in microwave for 3 minutes in a large glass measuring cup. Remove and add herbs (lavender or rosemary are excellent). Pour into a sterilized bottle.

Mint: Bruise a handful of mint leaves by rolling them with a pastry rolling pin. Pack them into a jar, and cover with apple cider vinegar. Let stand 2 weeks, then strain out mint. Pour remaining liquid in an empty, clean jar.

Rosewater: Mix the following in a jar: 1 pint apple cider vinegar, 1 ounce rose petals, $1/_2$ pint rosewater, $1/_2$ pint vinegar, and 1 ounce aromatic flowers such as sweet violet, rosemary, or lavender. Steep for 2 weeks, then strain. Pour remaining liquid in an empty, clean jar.

For thousands of years, human beings (especially women) have tried to change or improve their appearance by applying cosmetics—sometimes with deadly results. In the old world, limited scientific knowledge prevented awareness that many toxic and lethal chemicals were constantly being coated on people's skin in the name of good looks. Women in Roman Britain used a tin-oxide cream to whiten their faces. In 1558, Queen Elizabeth I began a fad by doing the same with egg whites, vinegar, and white powdered lead, a deadly mixture that caused poisoning and, ironically, scarring. By the 1700s, black "beauty spot" patches to cover the scars became necessary accessories.

SOLUTIONS FOR ACNE

Use a clean travel-size bottle to mix 1 teaspoon vinegar and 10 teaspoons water. Clean your face as usual in the morning, then carry this bottle and a few cotton balls with you so you can dab acne spots several times during the day. This solution shouldn't dry out your skin, and the vinegar will help return your skin to a natural pH balance. The treatment may also help prevent future acne outbreaks. Discontinue use if irritation worsens.

Make a paste of honey, wheat flour, and vinegar, then use it to lightly cover a new outbreak of pimples. Keep paste on overnight, and rinse off in the morning. This should enhance the healing process.

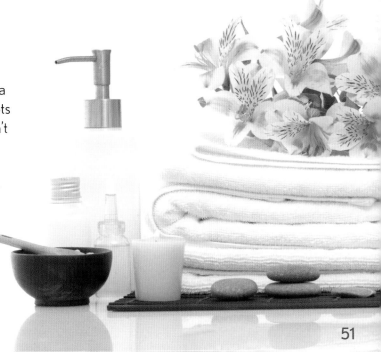

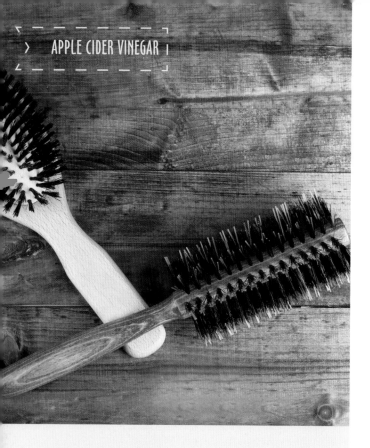

HAIR CARE

Vinegar is a great hair conditioner and can improve cleanliness and shine. For simple conditioning, just add 1 tablespoon vinegar to your hair as you rinse it.

Before shampooing, briefly soak hair in a small basin of water with ¼ cup apple cider vinegar added. Repeat several times a week to help control dandruff and remove buildup from sprays, shampoos, and conditioners.

Give your hair a conditioning treatment that will leave it feeling like you've been to an expensive salon. Mix together 3 eggs, 2 tablespoons olive oil or safflower oil, and 1 teaspoon vinegar, then apply to hair. Cover with a plastic cap, and leave on for a half hour. Shampoo as usual.

To control dandruff, mix 2 cups water and ½ cup vinegar, and use this to rinse after shampooing. If you need a stronger treatment for dandruff control, use this same method, but keep rinse on your hair for 1 hour, covered with a shower cap. Rinse. This mixture will also help control frizziness in dry or damaged hair.

Use 1 tablespoon apple cider vinegar mixed with 1 gallon water as an after-shampoo rinse to minimize gray in your hair.

This hair rinse can cover gray and treat dandruff at the same time. Combine 2 cups fresh sage and 1 cup fresh rosemary leaves in a pan, then add just enough water to cover the herbs. Bring mixture to a boil. Simmer for 6 hours, taking care not to let all the water boil away. Remove from heat, and let mixture steep overnight. Strain, then add enough water to make 5 cups. Add 2 teaspoons apple cider vinegar, and store in a plastic bottle. To use, thoroughly rub mixture into scalp, then lightly rinse.

Vinegar can help control an infestation of head lice. First use a medicated head lice shampoo, or follow your doctor's instructions for lice control. After shampooing hair, rinse with white vinegar, and go through hair with a comb dipped in vinegar. The vinegar will help loosen any remaining nits, or eggs, from hair. Continue with treatment prescribed on shampoo bottle.

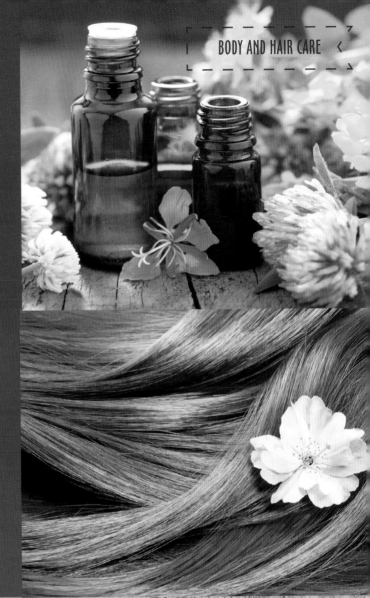

HERBAL RINSES

After you've shampooed your hair, give it added luster by conditioning with an herbal rinse. To make a rinse, add 3 tablespoons of dried or fresh herbs to a pint of boiling water. Steep for half an hour, strain and cool, and add ¼ cup apple cider vinegar.

RINSE FOR BLONDES

Steep 2 tablespoons of dried or fresh chamomile flowers and 1 tablespoon dried or fresh calendula flowers in 1 pint hot water for 30 minutes. Strain and cool. Add ¼ cup apple cider vinegar.

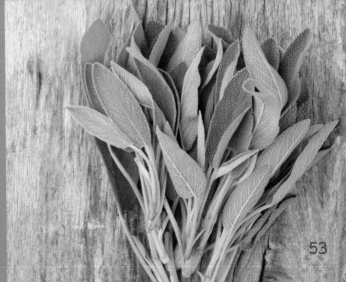

RINSE FOR BRUNETTES

To burnish darker-colored hair, substitute sage and rosemary for the chamomile and calendula in the recipe above.

53

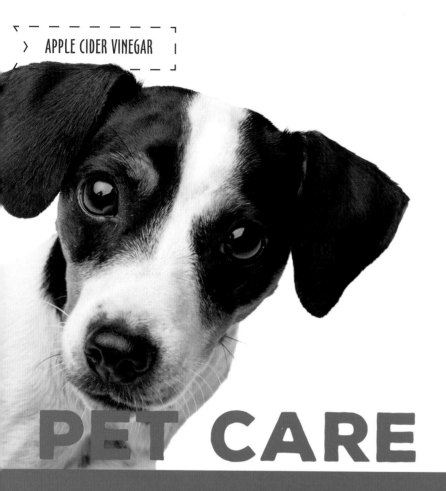
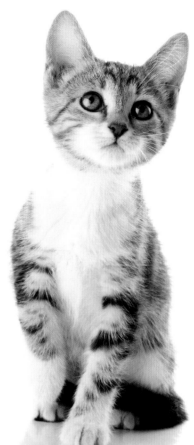

PET CARE

Don't keep the benefits of apple cider vinegar to yourself! Share them with your furry friends with these traditional remedies and healthful tips.

DOGS

Add 1 tablespoon apple cider vinegar to your dog's water bowl to improve overall health and digestion.

After a therapeutic shampoo to treat a skin infection, rinse dog with a solution of 1 part apple cider vinegar to 3 parts water.

Using vinegar as an after-shampoo treatment can make a dog's itchy skin feel better and his coat look shinier. Mix ½ cup vinegar into 1 gallon water, and coat dog's hair with solution. Leave it on coat for 10 minutes, then rinse thoroughly. Be sure to keep shampoo out of dog's eyes during this treatment.

CATS

Use vinegar to clean out a kitty litter pan. Remove litter, and pour in ½ inch vinegar. Let vinegar stand 15 minutes. Pour out, and thoroughly dry the pan. Then sprinkle with baking soda, and add fresh kitty litter.

If you're trying to keep your cats from walking on, sleeping on, or scratching certain items in your home, lightly sprinkle items with vinegar. The smell will keep cats away.

Add 1 tablespoon apple cider vinegar to your cat's water bowl to improve overall health and digestion.

CHICKENS

Use white or apple cider vinegar to clean out a chicken's water container. Pour vinegar directly onto a rag and wipe containers, then rinse with water.

HORSES

An apple a day keeps the flies away: Pour ¼ cup apple cider vinegar onto a horse's regular grain feed once a day to deter flies.

Spruce up a horse's coat by adding ½ cup vinegar to 1 quart water. Use this mixture in a spray bottle to apply to the horse's coat before showing.

HOMEMADE HORSE TREATS

Feed homemade treats to your horse, and you'll know what he's getting. Here's a recipe that will make a large quantity of nibbles to keep on hand. In large bowl, mix 1 cup molasses; ½ cup brown sugar; 4 large carrots, shredded; 1 cup finely chopped apples; and ½ cup apple cider vinegar. In another bowl, mix 2 cups bran, 1 cup sweet feed, and 1 cup flaxseed. Slowly add molasses mixture to dry ingredients until a dough forms. If dough is too thick, add more vinegar. If it becomes runny, add more bran. Drop batter onto a cookie sheet lined with aluminum foil, using a tablespoon. Flatten each piece of dough slightly, then bake at 300ºF for 1 hour. Turn cookies over with a spatula, and continue baking until they are completely dried, about another 45 minutes. Allow cookies to cool before feeding. Store in an airtight container.

Some arachnid collectors take great pride in adding a Giant Vinegaroon, a member of the whipscorpion family, to their collection. These 6-inch creatures look pretty nasty, but their main mode of defense is giving off a vinegar-scented acid from one of their glands. The acid won't generally harm people unless they are allergic to it, but a Vinegaroon's pinchers can do some damage. Some people keep them as pets, but you generally won't encounter one by chance because it hides by day and hunts at night. This creepy-looking arachnid is found only in the south and southwestern regions of the United States.

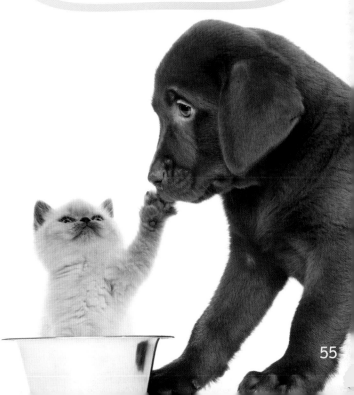

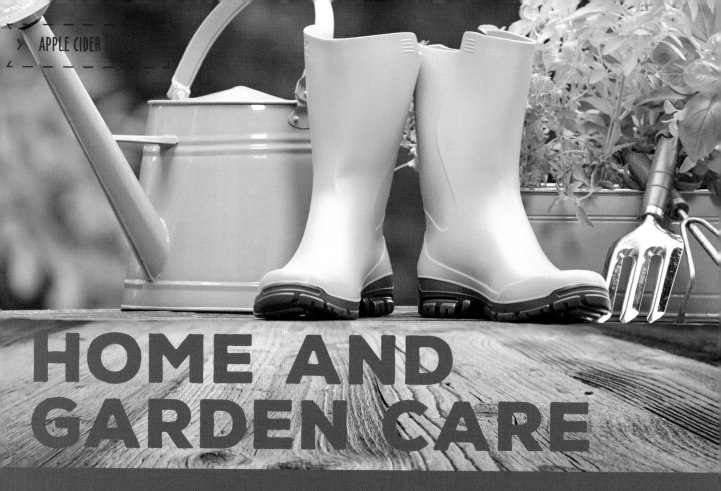

HOME AND GARDEN CARE

Rather than use harsh chemical products for cleaning and garden care, see what vinegar can do! Note that for cleaning, distilled white vinegar is often the best choice, unless otherwise specified.

CLEANING

For everyday cleaning of tile and grout, rub with a little apple cider vinegar on a sponge. This gives off a pleasant scent and will help cut any greasy buildup.

A bathtub ring requires a strong solvent. Try soaking paper towels with undiluted vinegar and placing them on the ring. Let towels dry out, then spray the tub with straight vinegar and scrub with a sponge.

Clean marble with a paste of baking soda and distilled white vinegar. Wipe clean and buff.

Mix equal amounts of white vinegar and water in a spray bottle. Spray onto mildewed areas and let sit for 15 minutes. Wipe clean. Use as a preventive measure in any area of your home that is prone to being damp, such as spaces under a sink or in the cellar.

Loosen up soap scum on shower doors and walls by spraying them with apple cider or white vinegar. Let dry, then respray to dampen. Wipe clean. Reapply and let sit for several hours. Then dampen and wipe clean again.

Shower curtains can become dulled by soap film or plagued with mildew. Keep vinegar in a spray bottle near your shower, and squirt shower curtains once or twice a week. No need to rinse.

For routine cleaning of sink and tub drains, pour in ½ cup baking soda followed by 1 cup distilled white vinegar. Let sit for 10 to 20 minutes, then flush with very hot water.

FLOWER CARE

Treat fresh-cut roses with extra care by displaying them in sterile vases with a preservative. Instead of a commercial preservative, mix 1 gallon water, 1 tablespoon vinegar, and 1 tablespoon granulated sugar. Flowers in a preservative solution will last about twice as long as those in plain water. You can also extend the lives of your flowers by replacing the water in the container every 2 to 3 days.

Another simple preservative for a vase of cut flowers is 1 quart warm water to which you've added 2 tablespoons vinegar and 1 teaspoon sugar.

Use this simple mixture to extend the life of your cut flowers: Mix 1 quart water, 1 tablespoon sugar, 1 teaspoon vinegar, and 1 teaspoon mouthwash.

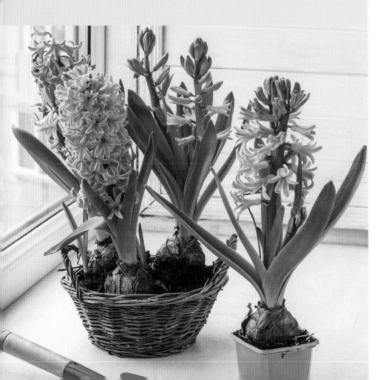

IN THE GARDEN

A squirt of vinegar may help invigorate a plant and make it more resistant to disease and pests. Mix 1 ounce vinegar with 1 gallon compost tea, and use as a regular spray on garden plants.

Combat plant diseases by combining 1 gallon vinegar, 1 cup orange oil, and 1 teaspoon Basic H or other mild soap. Spray solution on plants with your garden sprayer.

Mix 3 tablespoons natural apple cider vinegar in 1 gallon water. Fill garden sprayer with mixture, and spray roses daily to control black spot or other fungal diseases.

If seedlings begin to mold while starting them in a damp medium, clean them with a solution of 1 part vinegar to 9 parts water, and transfer to a new container. Spritz seeds regularly with this diluted mixture while awaiting germination.

To combat weeds, boil 1 quart water, then add 2 tablespoons salt and 5 tablespoons vinegar to it. While still hot, pour mixture directly onto weeds between cracks on sidewalks and driveways.

Fill a spray bottle with undiluted vinegar, and apply directly onto weeds or unwanted grass. You may have to repeat, but you should see weeds gradually wilt away.

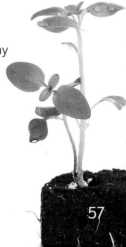

THE BENEFITS OF VINEGAR IN YOUR DIET

Apple cider vinegar is heralded as a potential healer of many of today's most common serious ailments. Devotees believe vinegar can help prevent or heal heart disease, diabetes, obesity, cancer, aging-related ailments, and a host of other conditions. They say it is full of vitamins, minerals, fiber, enzymes, and pectin and often attribute vinegar's medicinal effects to the presence of these ingredients.

The following are some of the specific claims made for apple cider vinegar:

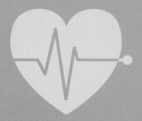

It reduces blood cholesterol levels and heart-disease risk. Apple cider vinegar fans say it contains pectin, which attaches to cholesterol and carries it out of the body, thus decreasing the risk of heart disease. In addition, many vinegar proponents say it is high in potassium, and high-potassium foods play a role in reducing the risk of heart disease by helping to prevent or lower high blood pressure. Calcium is also an important nutrient for keeping blood pressure in check, and vinegar is sometimes promoted as having a high calcium content. Many also claim vinegar helps the body absorb this essential mineral from other foods in the diet.

It treats diabetes. Apple cider vinegar may help control blood sugar levels, which helps to ward off diabetes complications, such as nerve damage and blindness. It also might help prevent other serious health problems, such as heart disease, that often go hand-in-hand with diabetes.

It fights obesity and aids in weight loss.
Some marketers proclaim that apple cider vinegar is high in fiber and therefore aids in weight loss. (Fiber provides bulk but is indigestible by the body, so foods high in fiber provide a feeling of fullness for fewer calories.)

A daily dose is also said to control or minimize the appetite. (Ironically, some folk traditions advise taking apple cider vinegar before a meal for the opposite effect—to stimulate the appetite in people who have lost interest in eating.)

It prevents cancer and aging. Apple cider vinegar proponents declare it contains high levels of the antioxidant beta-carotene (a form of vitamin A) and therefore helps prevent cancer and the ill effects of aging. (Antioxidants help protect the body's cells against damage from unstable molecules called free radicals; free-radical damage has been linked to various conditions, including coronary heart disease, cancer, and the aging process.)

It prevents osteoporosis. Advocates say apple cider vinegar releases calcium and other minerals from the foods you eat so your body is better able to absorb and use them to strengthen bones. Vinegar allegedly allows the body to absorb one-third more calcium from green vegetables than it would without the aid of vinegar. Some fans also say apple cider vinegar is itself a great source of calcium.

Based on these claims, apple cider vinegar certainly seems to be a wonder food. And it's understandably tempting to want to believe that some food or drug or substance will make diabetes,

obesity, cancer, and osteoporosis go away with little or no discomfort, effort, or risk.

However, as a wise consumer, you know that when something sounds too good to be true, it almost certainly is. So when it comes to your health—especially when you're dealing with such major medical conditions—it's important to take a step back and look carefully at the evidence.

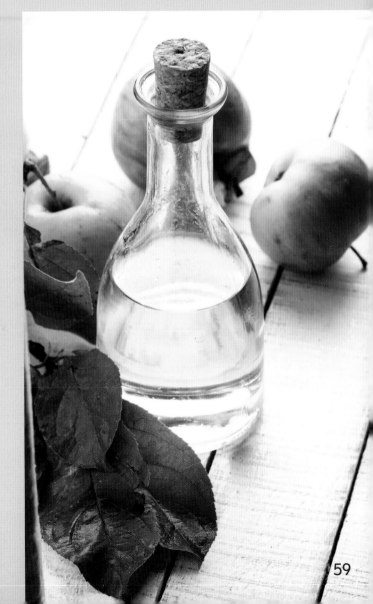

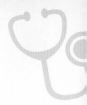

A CLOSER LOOK AT THE CLAIMS

With such dramatic claims made for it, you would think that vinegar would be high on the lists of medical researchers searching for the next break-through. Yet in the past 20 years, there has been very little research into the use of vinegar for thera-peutic health purposes.

Granted, a lack of supporting scientific research is a common problem with many natural and alterna-tive therapies. But even the National Center for Complementary and Alternative Medicine (NC-CAM), a division of the U.S. government's National Institutes of Health that was created specifically to investigate natural or unconventional therapies that hold promise, has not published any studies about vinegar, despite the fact that there has been re-newed interest in vinegar's healing benefits recently.

So without solid scientific studies, can we judge whether vinegar provides the kinds of dramatic benefits that its promoters and fans attribute to it? Not conclusively. But we can look at the claims and compare them to the little scientific knowledge we do have about vinegar.

Those who have faith in apple cider vinegar as a wide-ranging cure say its healing properties come from an abundance of nutrients that remain after apples are fermented to make apple cider vin-egar. They contend that vinegar is rich in minerals and vitamins, including calcium, potassium, and beta-carotene; complex carbohydrates and fiber, including the soluble fiber pectin; amino acids (the building blocks of protein); beneficial enzymes; and acetic acid (which gives vinegar its taste). These substances do play many important roles in

health and healing, and some are even considered essential nutrients for human health. The problem is that standard nutritional analysis of vinegar, including apple cider vinegar, has not shown it to be a good source of most of these substances.

Take a look at the table on pages 61–62—it shows the results of a nutritional analysis of an apple com-pared with the nutritional breakdown of two different amounts of apple cider vinegar. One tablespoon of apple cider vinegar per day is the typical therapeutic dose recommended, so the nutrients found in this amount of the vinegar are shown in the second col-umn of the table. Just to be sure that the small amount of vinegar in a tablespoon isn't the sole explanation for the apparent lack of nutrients, the table also in-cludes the nutritional analysis of a larger amount (half a cup) of vinegar. You'll notice that even at that higher dose, vinegar does not appear to include significant amounts of most of the nutrients that are claimed to be the source of its medicinal value.

To put all this information into some context, the column at the far right in the table shows the daily amounts needed by a typical adult who con-sumes 2,000 calories per day. (Re-quirements haven't been established for some of the other substances that are often cited as contributing to vinegar's beneficial effects.)

As you can see, the one milligram of calcium in one tablespoon of apple cider vinegar does not come close to the 300 milligrams of calcium in eight

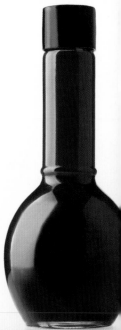

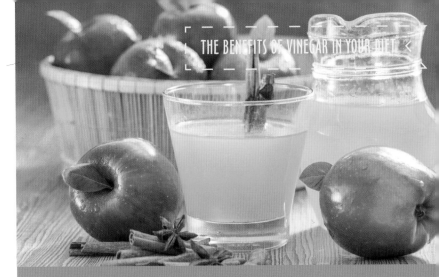

ounces of milk, as some promoters of apple cider vinegar claim. In fact, it supplies only a tiny fraction of the 1,000 milligrams a typical adult needs in a day. Vinegar also contains little potassium.

In terms of pectin, the type of soluble fiber that is said to bind to cholesterol and help carry it out of the body, apple cider vinegar contains no measurable amounts of it or of any other type of fiber. So it would seem that pectin could not account for any cholesterol-binding activity that vinegar might be shown to have.

Do apple cider vinegar's secrets lie in the vitamins it contains? No. According to the USDA, apple cider vinegar contains no vitamin A, vitamin B 6 , vitamin C, vitamin E, vitamin K, thiamin, riboflavin, niacin, pantothenic acid, or folate.

What about some of the other health-boosting substances that are alleged to be in vinegar? According to detailed nutritional analyses, apple cider vinegar contains no significant amounts of amino acids. Nor does it contain ethyl alcohol, caffeine, theobromine, beta-carotene, alpha-carotene, beta-crypto-xanthin, lycopene, lutein, or zeaxanthin.

Nutrient	One medium apple, raw (2¾ inch diameter)	1 Tbsp. apple cider vinegar	½ cup apple cider vinegar	Daily amount needed by avg. adult
Calories	72	3	25	2,000
Carbohydrate	19.06 g	0.14 g	1.11 g	130 g
Fat	0.23 g	0 g	0 g	65 g (max.)
Protein	0.36 g	0 g	0 g	46 g (women) 56 g (men)
Fiber	3.3 g	0 g	0 g	25 g (women) 38 g (men)
MINERALS				
Calcium	8 mg	1 mg	8 mg	1,000 mg
Iron	0.17 mg	0.03 mg	0.24 mg	18 mg (women) 8 g (men)

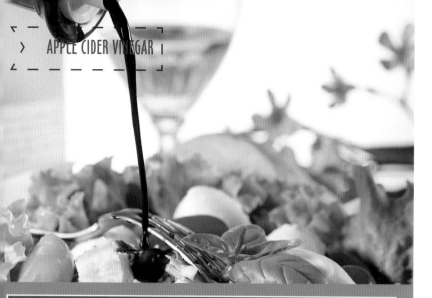

Nutrient	One medium apple, raw (2 3/4 inch diameter)	1 Tbsp. apple cider vinegar	1/2 cup apple cider vinegar	Daily amount needed by avg. adult
Magnesium	7 mg	1 mg	6 mg	320 g (women) 420 g (men)
Phosphorus	15 mg	1 mg	10 mg	700 mg
Potassium	148 mg	11 mg	87 mg	4,700 mg
Sodium	1 mg	1 mg	6 mg	1,500 mg
Zinc	0.06 mg	0.01 mg	0.05 mg	8 mg (women) 11 mg (men)
Copper	0.037 mg	0.001 mg	0.01 mg	900 mcg
Manganese	0.048 mg	0.037 mg	0.298 mg	1.8 mg (women) 2.3 mg (men)
Selenium	0 mcg	0 mcg	0.1 mcg	55 mcg

HOW VINEGAR CAN HELP

So if vinegar doesn't actually contain all the substances that are supposed to account for its medicinal benefits, does that mean it has no healing powers? Hardly. As mentioned, so little research has been done on vinegar that we can't totally rule out many of the dramatic claims made it.

Although we know vinegar doesn't contain loads of nutrients traditionally associated with good health, it may well contain yet-to-be-identified phytochemicals (beneficial compounds in plants) that would account for some of the healing benefits that vinegar fans swear by. Scientists continue to discover such beneficial substances in all kinds of foods.

But beyond that possibility, there appear to be more tangible and realistic—albeit less sensational—ways that vinegar can help the body heal. Rather than being the dramatic blockbuster cure that we are endlessly (and fruitlessly) searching for, vinegar seems quite capable of playing myriad supporting roles—as part of an overall lifestyle approach—that can help us fight serious health conditions, such as osteoporosis, diabetes, and heart disease.

INCREASING CALCIUM ABSORPTION

If there is one thing vinegar fans, marketers, alternative therapists, and scientists alike can agree on, it's that vinegar is high in acetic acid. And acetic acid, like other acids, can increase the body's absorption of important minerals from the foods we eat. Therefore, including apple cider vinegar in meals or possibly even drinking a mild tonic of vinegar and water (up to a tablespoon of vinegar in a glass of water) just before or with meals might improve your body's ability to absorb the essential minerals locked in foods.

Vinegar may be especially useful to women, who generally have a hard time getting all the calcium their bodies need to keep bones strong and prevent the debilitating, bone-thinning disease osteoporosis. Although dietary calcium is most abundant in dairy products such as milk, many women (and men) suffer from a condition called lactose intolerance that makes it difficult or impossible for them to digest the sugar in milk. As a result, they may suffer uncomfortable gastrointestinal symptoms, such as cramping and diarrhea, when they consume dairy products. These women must often look elsewhere to fulfill their dietary calcium needs.

Dark, leafy greens are good sources of calcium, but some of these greens also contain compounds that inhibit calcium absorption. Fortunately for dairy-deprived women (and even those who do drink milk), a few splashes of vinegar or a tangy vinaigrette on their greens may very well allow them to absorb more valuable calcium.

CONTROLLING BLOOD SUGAR LEVELS

Vinegar has recently won attention for its potential to help people with type 2 diabetes get a better handle on their disease. Improved control could help them delay or prevent such complications as blindness, impotence, and a loss of feeling in the extremities that may necessitate amputation.

Also, because people with diabetes are at increased risk for other serious health problems, such as heart disease, improved control of their diabetes could potentially help to ward off these associated conditions, as well.

With type 2 diabetes, the body's cells become resistant to the action of the hormone insulin. The body normally releases insulin into the bloodstream in response to a meal. Insulin's job is to help the body's cells take in the glucose, or sugar, from the carbohydrates in food, so they can use it for energy.

But when the body's cells become insulin resistant, sugar from food begins to build up in the blood, even while the cells themselves are starving for it. (High levels of insulin tend to build up in the blood, too, because the body releases more and more insulin to try to transport the large amounts of sugar out of the bloodstream and into the cells.)

Over time, high levels of blood sugar can damage nerves throughout the body and otherwise cause irreversible harm. So one major goal of diabetes treatment is to normalize blood sugar levels and keep them in a healthier range as much as possible. And that's where vinegar appears to help.

It seems that vinegar may be able to inactivate some of the digestive enzymes that break the carbohydrates from food into sugar, thus slowing the absorption of sugar from a meal into the bloodstream. Slowing sugar absorption gives the insulin-resistant body more time to pull sugar out of the blood and thus helps prevent the blood sugar level from rising so high. Blunting the sudden jump in blood sugar that would usually occur after a meal also lessens the

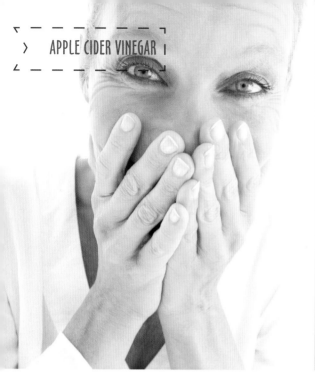
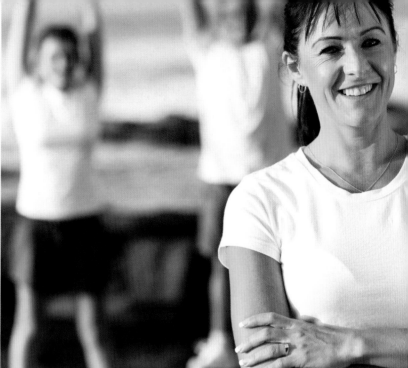

amount of insulin the body needs to release at one time to remove the sugar from the blood.

A study cited in 2004 in the American Diabetes Association's publication *Diabetes Care* indicates that vinegar holds real promise for helping people with diabetes. In the study, 21 people with either type 2 diabetes or insulin resistance (a prediabetic condition) and 8 control subjects were each given a solution containing five teaspoons of vinegar, five teaspoons of water, and one teaspoon of saccharin two minutes before ingesting a high-carbohydrate meal. The blood sugar and insulin levels of the participants were measured before the meal and 30 minutes and 60 minutes after the meal.

Vinegar increased overall insulin sensitivity 34 percent in the study participants who were insulin-resistant and 19 percent in those with type 2 diabetes. That means their bodies actually became more receptive to insulin, allowing the hormone to do its job of getting sugar out of the blood and into the cells. Both blood sugar and blood insulin levels were lower than usual in the insulin-resistant participants, which is more good news. Surprisingly, the control group (who had neither diabetes nor a prediabetic condition but were given the vinegar solution) also experienced a reduction in insulin levels in the blood. These findings are significant because, in addition to the nerve damage caused by perpetually elevated blood sugar levels, several chronic conditions, including heart disease, have been linked to excess insulin in the blood over prolonged periods of time.

More studies certainly need to be done to confirm the extent of vinegar's benefits for type 2 diabetes patients and those at risk of developing this increasingly common disease. But for now, people with type 2 diabetes might be wise to talk with their doctors or dietitians about consuming more vinegar.

REPLACING UNHEALTHY FATS AND SODIUM

There are some delicious varieties of vinegar available—and you're not limited to apple cider vinegar to get the benefits! Each bestows a different taste or character on foods. The diversity and intensity of flavor are key to one important healing role that vinegar can play. Whether you are trying to protect yourself from cardiovascular diseases, such as heart disease, high blood pressure, or stroke, or you have been diagnosed with one or more of these conditions and have been advised to clean up your diet, vinegar should become a regular cooking and dining companion.

That's because a tasty vinegar can often be used in place of sodium and/or ingredients high in saturated or trans fats to add flavor and excitement to a variety of dishes.

Saturated and trans fats have been shown to have a detrimental effect on blood cholesterol levels, and experts recommend that people who have or are at risk of developing high blood pressure cut back on the amount of sodium they consume. Using vinegar as a simple, flavorful substitute for these less healthful ingredients as often as possible can help people manage blood cholesterol and blood pressure levels and, in turn, help ward off heart disease and stroke.

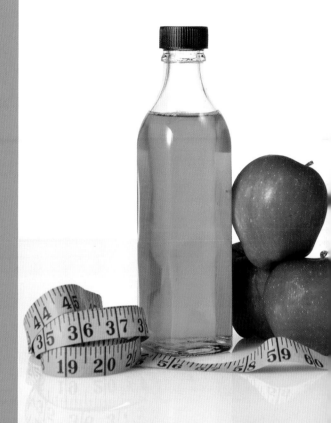

The suggestions on the next page will give you some sense of how vinegar can help you create and enjoy a diet that may lower your blood cholesterol and blood pressure and decrease your risks of heart disease and stroke.

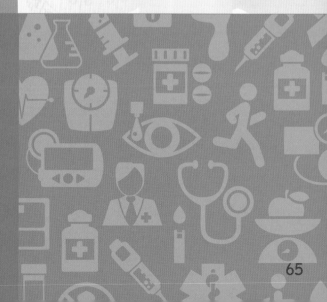

65

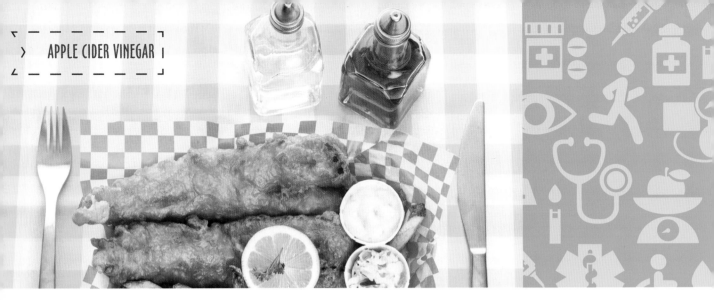

• Make a vinegar-based coleslaw rather than a creamy, mayonnaise-based one. Because mayonnaise is made up almost completely of unhealthy fats and cholesterol, this easy switch can dramatically reduce the cholesterol and fat in this popular side dish.

• Enjoy healthier fish and chips. Instead of dipping fish in tartar sauce and drenching fries in salt and ketchup, splash them with a little malt vinegar. (Also consider baking the fish and the potatoes instead of frying them.) Because it contains mayonnaise, tartar sauce is high in unhealthy fats and cholesterol.

•Use vinegar-based salad dressings instead of creamy, mayonnaise-based dressings. Choose or make a flavorful herb salad dressing that contains mostly water, vinegar, and just a touch of oil to help it adhere to your salad veggies.

• Opt for vinegar instead of mayonnaise or other common, bad-fat-laden sandwich spreads to add flavor and moisture to sandwiches.

• When making a dish that contains beans, add a little vinegar near the end of cooking—it will dramatically decrease the amount of salt you'll need. It perks up the flavor of beans without raising your blood pressure.

• You can also use vinegar as a tangy marinade for tenderizing less-fatty cuts of meat. Choosing meat with less fat on the edges and less marbling within is one of the easiest ways to trim unhealthy fats from your diet. Unfortunately, meats that don't have as much marbling tend to be a little tougher. So vinegar can do double duty by adding a dash of zing as it tenderizes.

ADDING EXCITEMENT TO A HEALTHY DIET

Some of our strongest natural weapons against cancer and aging are fruits and vegetables. The antioxidants and phytochemicals they contain seem to hold real promise in lowering our risk of many types of cancer. Their antioxidants also help to protect cells from the free-radical damage that is thought to underlie many of the changes we associate with aging. Protected cells don't wear out and need replacing as often as cells that aren't bathed in antioxidants. Scientists think this continual cell replacement may be at the root of aging.

It is recommended that the average person eat about two cups of fruit and two-and-a-half cups of vegetables every day. One way to add excitement and variety to all those vegetables is to use vinegar liberally as a seasoning.

> Vinegar loses some of its pungency when heated. If you want to enjoy vinegar's full tart taste, add it to a dish at the end of cooking. Also, after heating up leftovers, splash them with vinegar to perk up their flavors.

• Rice vinegar and a little soy sauce give veggies an Asian flavor or can form the base of an Asian coleslaw.

• Red wine vinegar or white wine vinegar can turn boring vegetables into a quick-and-easy marinated-vegetable salad that's ready to be grabbed out of the refrigerator whenever hunger strikes. Just chop your favorite veggies, put them in a bowl with a marinade of vinegar, herbs, and a dash of olive oil, and let them sit for at least an hour. (You don't need much oil to make the marinade stick to the veggies, so go light, and be sure you choose olive oil.)

• Toss chopped vegetables in a vinegar-and-olive-oil salad dressing before loading them on skewers and putting them on the backyard grill. The aroma and flavor will actually have your family asking for seconds—of vegetables!

• After steaming vegetables, drizzle a little of your favorite vinegar over them instead of adding butter or salt. They'll taste so good, you may never get to the meat on your plate.

• By enhancing the flavor of vegetables with vinegar, you and your family will be inclined to eat more of them. And that—many researchers and doctors would agree—will likely go a long way toward protecting your body's cells from the damage that can lead to cancer and other problems of aging.

• When poaching fish, put a tablespoon of vinegar in the poaching water to keep the fish from falling apart. Vinegar helps the protein in the fish coagulate, and mushiness isn't a problem because fish is usually poached for less than 20 minutes.

• When a recipe calls for buttermilk and you have none, substitute plain milk and add a little apple cider vinegar. Use one table-spoon of vinegar per cup (eight ounces) of milk. Let stand 10 to 15 minutes at room temperature until it thickens, then use it in your recipe as you would buttermilk. Mild-flavored vinegars such as apple cider vinegar are best for this purpose.

• Cover peeled potatoes with water and a tablespoon or two of vinegar to keep them from browning.

In 1756, the duc de Richelieu invented the recipe for mayonnaise with his particular mixture of egg yolks, vinegar, oil, and seasonings. The name may have come from a town in Minorca, an island off of Spain.

REMOVING HARMFUL SUBSTANCES FROM PRODUCE

Some people are concerned that eating large amounts of fruits and vegetables may lead to an unhealthy consumption of pesticides and other farm-chemical residues. Vinegar can lend a hand here, too. Washing produce in a mixture of water and vinegar appears to help remove certain pesticides, according to the small amount of research that has been published. Vinegar also appears to be helpful in getting rid of harmful bacteria on fruits and vegetables.

To help remove potentially harmful residues, mix a solution of 10 percent vinegar to 90 percent water (for example,

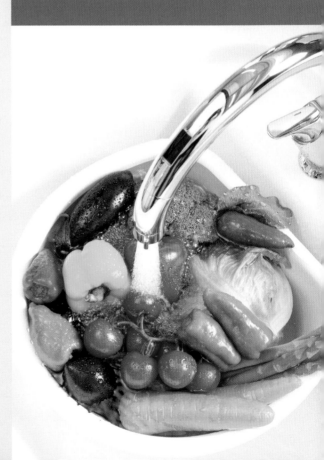

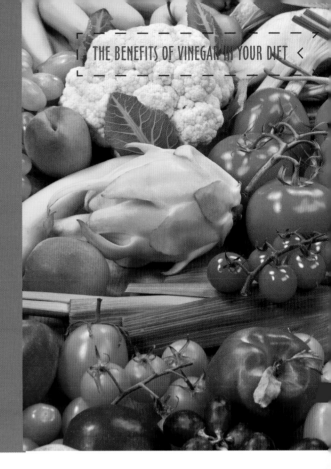

mix one cup of white vinegar in nine cups of water). Then, place produce in the vinegar solution, let it soak briefly, and then swish it around in the solution. Finally, rinse the produce thoroughly.

Do not use this process on tender, fragile fruits, such as berries, that might be damaged in the process or soak up too much vinegar through their porous skins. Some pesticide residues are trapped beneath the waxy coatings that are applied to certain vegetables to help them retain moisture. The vinegar solution probably won't wash those pesticides away, so peeling lightly may be a better option. Some research suggests that cooking further eliminates some pesticide residue.

ADDING FLAVOR, NOT CALORIES

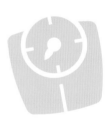

Vinegar contains very few calories—only 25 in half a cup! Compare that to the nearly 800 calories you get in half a cup of mayonnaise, and you have a real fat-fighting food. So if you're looking to lose weight, using vinegar in place of mayonnaise whenever you can will help you make a serious dent in your calorie (and fat) intake.

Vinegar can also help you have your dessert and cut calories, too. Use a splash of balsamic vinegar to bring out the sweetness and flavor of strawberries without any added sugar. Try it on other fruits that you might sprinkle sugar on—you'll be pleasantly surprised at the difference a bit of balsamic vinegar can make. And for a real unexpected treat on a hot summer evening, drizzle balsamic vinegar—instead of high-fat, sugary caramel or chocolate sauce—on a dish of reduced-fat vanilla ice cream. Can't imagine that combination? Just try it.

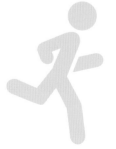

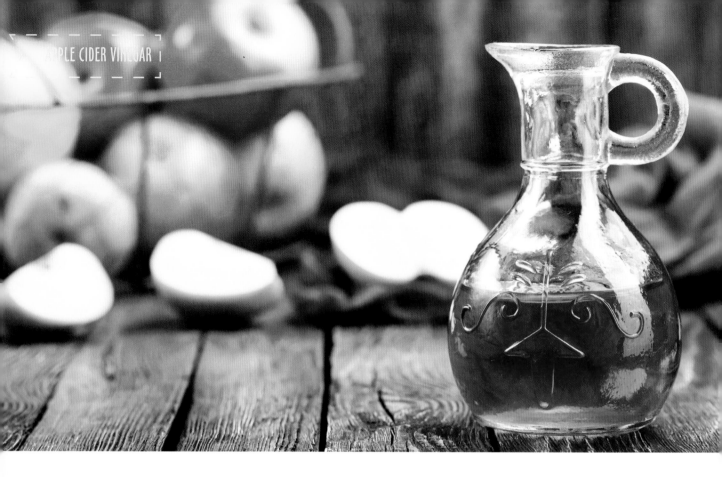

SHOULD YOU SUPPLEMENT?

Some people believe in the healing power of apple cider vinegar but would rather take it in tablet form instead of using it as a daily tonic or adding it to food.

But like any shortcut on the road to better health, you can't be sure this one will get you to the goal you're aiming for.

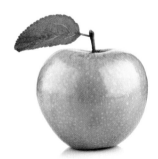

Part of the reason for concern is that the U.S. Food and Drug Administration (FDA) does not regulate supplements, so you really can't be sure what you're getting. In a study reported in the July 2005 *Journal of the American Dietetic Association*, for example, researchers analyzed eight different brands of apple cider vinegar tablets. The analysis showed most had acetic acid levels different from those claimed on the label. How much of a problem is this? Well, it would be natural to think the more acetic acid the better. But in truth, at a level of 11 percent, acetic acid can cause burns to the skin. And at 20 percent, it is considered poisonous. Some of the analyzed supplements, however, claimed to contain a frightening 35 percent acetic acid! Fortunately for their users, none did. The

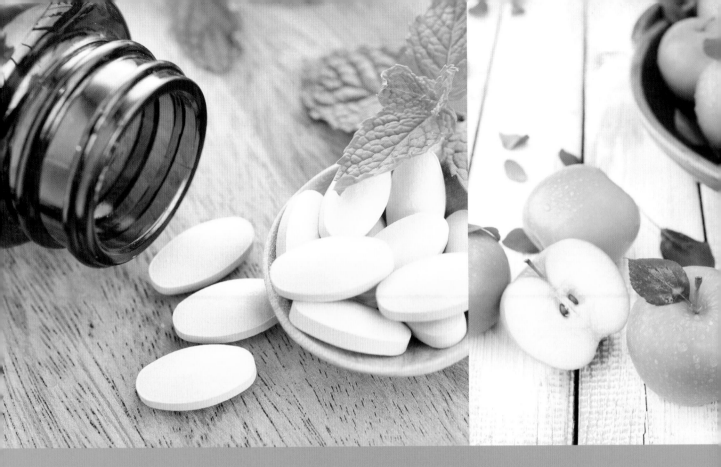

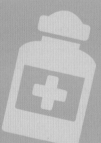

acetic acid content actually ranged from 1.04 percent to 10.57 percent. Another reason to go natural: Several of the samples were contaminated with mold and/ or yeast, including one that claimed to be yeast-free. In addition, because so little scientific research has been done to verify the healing claims made for vinegar— and the possible ingredients or actions that might be responsible—it's impossible to know if supplements would have the same effects as the real thing. Indeed, most of vinegar's benefits—at least the ones that rest on the most solid scientific grounds—are those based on its use as a substitute for unhealthy ingredients in the diet, a role that simply could not be played by a pill.

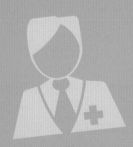

So at this time, it would seem you are almost certainly better off including more vinegar in your diet, taking advantage of its potential healing benefits as well as its phenomenal flavors, rather than spending more money on supplements that may not have any benefit and could even be dangerous.

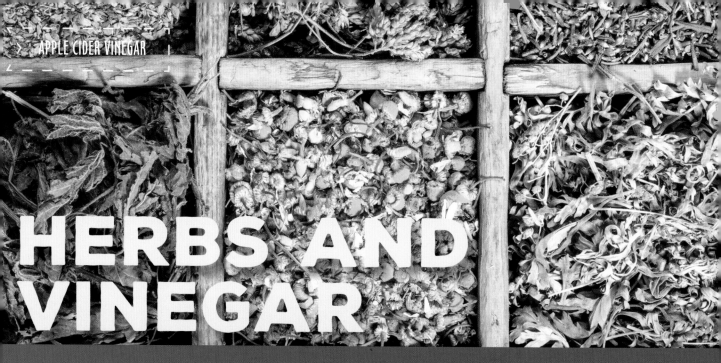

HERBS AND VINEGAR

Herbs have long intrigued us—and for good reason. Because of their potential as food and as medicine, they have been seen as a valuable resource for humans throughout the ages. In this chapter we'll look at some herbs that pair very well with vinegar, offering good taste, nourishment, and healing. You may even find yourself growing your own herbs or making your own herbal remedies!

VINEGAR OF THE FOUR THIEVES

Here's a recipe handed down from the Middle Ages. Herbal lore has it that four men caught ransacking empty homes infested with bubonic plague were tried before a court in Marseilles. Asked by the judge how the men had avoided contracting the plague, the accused men said they had washed themselves with a special herbal vinegar. The thieves were granted freedom in return for the recipe.

You can add this vinegar to a bath, or take 1 teaspoon internally——no more than 1 tablespoon an hour——to protect yourself during flu season.

2	quarts apple cider vinegar
2	Tbsp lavender
2	Tbsp rosemary
2	Tbsp sage
2	Tbsp wormwood
2	Tbsp rue
2	Tbsp mint
2	Tbsp garlic buds, unpeeled

Cover the herbs with vinegar. Keep at room temperature for two weeks. Strain and bottle. You can also make a vinegar syrup by adding 4 ounces of glycerine. Sweeten to taste.

GATHERING HERBS

Gathering plants you've grown yourself gives you a tremendous sense of accomplishment, but you may also collect herbs growing wild. Gathering herbs from the wild is referred to as "wildcrafting." If you pick wild herbs, however, be certain you've identified them properly. Some poisonous herbs resemble harmless ones. Also, make sure the area where you're wildcrafting is free of pesticides, chemical sprays, or other pollutants. Avoid picking herbs growing along busy roads or highways where car exhaust can contaminate them. Do not harvest rare or endangered plants from the wild. Many plant species are threatened through both overharvesting and loss of habitat. Cultivating herbs yourself can help preserve the native habitats of some endangered plant species.

HARVESTING YOUR HERBS

As a general rule, harvest the leaves of an herb when the plant is about to flower—usually in the spring or fall. (Plants are very high in volatile oils right before they flower.) Harvest roots and bark in the fall and winter months when the plant is dormant and its nutrients are in storage.

Gather herbs in the morning on a dry day. Herbs that are dry when harvested are less likely to mold or spoil during processing. Avoid washing leaves and flowers of herbs after you've harvested them. If the herbs are covered with dirt or dust, rinse them off with a garden hose or watering can, then allow the herbs to dry for a day or two before picking them. When wildcrafting, shake the water off wet herbs; you may also try drying wild herbs by gently blotting them with a towel. The root of the herb is the only part of that plant you should wash thoroughly after harvesting.

Harvesting the seeds of an herb requires a little more intuition. You need to check your plants everyday, and be prepared to harvest the seeds as soon as you notice they've begun to dry. (Timing is crucial: You must allow the seeds to ripen, but catch them before they fall off the plant.) Carefully snap off seed heads over a large paper bag, allowing the seeds to fall into it. Leave the seeds in the bag until they have dried completely.

DRYING HERBS

Herbal preparations often require the use of dried herbs. To dry herbs, hang them upside down until they are crisp. If you have a spare countertop or closet shelf, you can spread the herbs over newspaper or paper towels. (Keep the herbs evenly distributed, avoiding thick, wet piles.) Cover the herbs with a paper towel or a very thin piece of cheesecloth to prevent dust from settling.

Do not dry herbs in direct sunlight. Dry herbs in an area that is hot, well ventilated, and free of moisture, such as a barn, loft, or covered porch. In these conditions, the moisture will evaporate quickly from the plants, but the aromatic oils will remain in the leaves.

You can also use a food dehydrator (use the lowest setting) to dry your herbs. If you're handy with a saw and hammer and nails, you can build a drying cabinet in which the herbs sit on screens and warm air circulates through the screens. A drying cabinet can be a plain cupboard in a warm, dry location, or it can be a fancy version with a solar or electric heater with fans to circulate the air. Whatever drying method you use, the optimal temperature for drying herbs is approximately 85 degrees Fahrenheit. Higher temperatures can harm the herbs and dissipate the volatile oils.

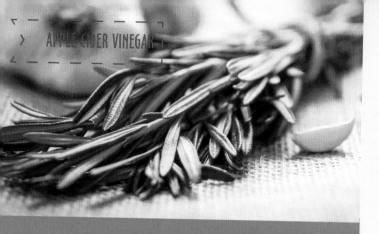

It may take up to a week to dry some herbs, depending on the thickness of the plant's leaves and stem. As soon as leaves are fully dry—but before they become brittle—strip them from the stems. Store the leaves immediately in airtight containers to preserve their flavor and aroma. Label the containers with the herb name and date stored.

STORING HERBS

Once you've fully dried your herbs, don't delay in storing them in airtight containers or your herbs will lose essential oils. Simply crumble the herbs before storing. Avoid grinding and powdering herbs because they won't retain their flavor as long.

Glass jars with tight-sealing lids or glass stoppers are ideal for storing dried herbs. You may also use porcelain canisters that close tightly, plastic pill holders with tight covers, and sealable plastic bags, buckets, or barrels for large herb pieces.

Store herbs in a dark place to preserve their color and flavor. If you must store herbs in a lighted area, keep them in dark-colored jars that block out most of the light. The worst place to keep herbs is in a spice rack over the stove: Heat from cooking will cause your herbs to lose their flavor quickly. Remember to label each container, including its contents and date of harvest.

MAKING HERBAL MEDICINES AND PREPARATIONS

You've grown your herbs, gathered them, and dried them. The next step is to prepare them. Preparing herbs is simple and easy—not to mention economical.

The goal of the herbalist is to release the volatile oils, antibiotics, aromatics, and other healing chemicals an herb contains. Among other preparation methods such as capsules and poultices, you can soak herbs in vinegar to produce long-lasting tinctures.

FIRST STEPS

Lay out all the cooking, storage, and labeling materials you'll need to prepare your herbal home remedies. Don't attempt to make salves, syrups, and tinctures all at once. Overly enthusiastic beginners often try to do too much too soon. Even the most experienced practitioner can get confused and make mistakes. Concentrate on making only one type of herbal remedy at a time.

Don't overharvest your herbs. Don't bring in a basketful of rosemary if the recipe calls for no more than an ounce. Think small when you store your herbs, too. Salves and other preparations tend to last longer when stored in small batches. If you intend to save these medicines for longer than a few months, tightly stopper bottles, seal jars with wax, and refrigerate liquid preparations.

TINCTURES

One popular way of making herbal medicines is to produce a tincture. Used for herbs that require a solvent stronger than water to release their chemical constituents, a tincture is an herb extracted in alcohol, glycerine, or vinegar. Vinegar, because it contains the solvent acetic acid, is an alternative to alcohol in tinctures—especially for herbs that are high in alkaloids, which require acids to dissolve. You can use herbal vinegars medicinally or dilute them with additional vinegar to make great-tasting salad dressings and marinades. Use any vinegar with herbs, but to keep your vinegars natural, you may wish to use apple cider vinegar. Apple cider vinegar is made by naturally fermenting apple juice, while white distilled vinegar is an industrial byproduct. Rice vinegar, red wine vinegar, and balsamic vinegar are also good choices, but they are a bit more expensive, and their strong flavors sometimes require additional herbs.

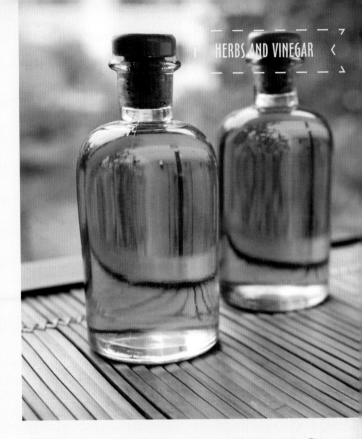

Tinctures can be added to hot or cold water to make an instant tea or mixed with water for external use in compresses and foot baths. The advantage of tinctures is that they have a long shelf life, and they're available for use in a pinch. You can even add tinctures to oils or salves to create instant healing ointments. You can apply a vinegar tincture to the skin to bring down a fever. Dilute the tincture with an equal amount of cool water. Soak a cloth in the solution and bathe the body. As the solution evaporates, it cools the body, often lowering the body's temperature by several degrees. Vinegar is also a potent antifungal agent and makes a good athlete's foot soak when combined with antifungal herbs.

With common kitchen utensils and very little effort, you can easily prepare suitable tinctures. First, clean and pick over fresh herbs, removing any insects or damaged plant material. Remove leaves and flowers from stems, and break roots or bark into smaller pieces. Of course, you can use dried herbs, too. Cut or chop the plant parts you want to process or chop in a blender or food processor. Cover with vinegar. Puree the plant material and transfer it to a glass jar. Make sure the vinegar covers the plants. Plant materials exposed to air can mold or rot, so add more vinegar if needed. This is especially important if you use fresh herbs. Store the jar at room temperature out of sunlight, and shake the jar everyday. After three to six weeks, strain the liquid with a kitchen strainer, cheesecloth, thin piece of muslin, or a paper coffee filter. Even when you've managed to strain out every last bit of plant material, sometimes more particles mysteriously show up after the tincture has been stored. There is no harm in using a tincture that contains a bit of solid debris. Tinctures will keep for many years without refrigeration.

Because the usual dosage of a tincture is 15 to 30 drops, you receive enough herb to benefit from its medicinal properties with very little vinegar.

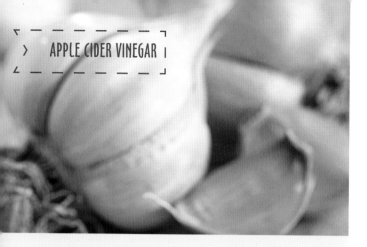

FOOT SOAK VINEGAR

Place two garlic bulbs in a blender along with two handfuls of fresh or dried calendula petals, one handful of chopped fresh comfrey root, and the chopped hulls of several black walnuts (or use ½ oz black walnut tincture). Pour vinegar over the herbs and blend well. Place mixture in a large, shallow pan, and add 20 drops of tea tree oil.

To treat athlete's foot, soak feet in the solution for at least 15 minutes. Rinse feet and dry in the sun or in the light of a sun lamp. Use the foot soak three to four times a day. Make a fresh batch of the mixture for each use.

KITCHEN VINEGAR

Not only does this preparation taste great in salads, stir-fries, and marinades, but it contains antibacterial properties as well. Gather fresh oregano and basil leaves and place in a blender with ten peeled cloves of garlic. Pour vinegar over the herbs and blend. Bottle and allow to sit for several weeks. Strain out the herbs or leave them in the preparation. For additional flavor and a nice presentation, you may add a whole sprig of oregano or basil, a cayenne pepper, and several lemon or orange rinds. This vinegar keeps well for several months unrefrigerated.

BASIL

Basil produces a neat, dense growth, with bright-green, triangular leaves. You can even clip basil into a neat hedge. A compact dwarf variety, Spicy Globe, makes an outstanding edging or an attractive container plant.

A member of the mint family, basil is recommended to aid digestion and expel gas. It's also good for treating stomach cramps, vomiting, and constipation. It has been found to be more effective than drugs to relieve nausea from chemotherapy and radiation.

Basil has a slight sedative action and sometimes is recommended for nervous headaches and anxiety. Studies show that extracts of basil seeds have antibacterial properties. Basil contains vitamins A and C as well as antioxidants, which prevent cell damage. One study found that basil increases production of disease-fighting antibodies up to 20 percent.

In the kitchen, basil's rich, spicy flavor—something like pepper with a hint of mint and cloves—works wonders in pesto, tomato sauce, salads, cheese dishes, eggs, stews, vinegars, and all sorts of vegetables. Often you'll find basil in ethnic cuisines, particularly those of Italy and Thailand.

USAGE

Take prunings and use fresh leaves any time. Harvest basil when buds are about to blossom—when the plant is at its flavor peak—and hang-dry. Basil retains its flavor best when frozen or stored in oil or vinegar.

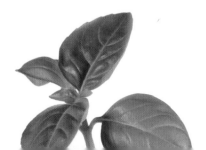

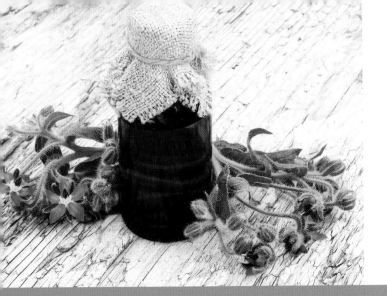

PRECAUTIONS

Borage is safe to use in moderation. Claims that it may harm the liver have not been substantiated, but you may want to limit how much you use; the herb contains the same type of alkaloids as comfrey. Some researchers strongly suggest not eating the leaves, which contain higher amounts of pyrrolizidine alkaloids than the flowers do.

BORAGE

Celtic warriors drank borage wine because they believed it gave them courage. Romans thought borage produced a sense of elation and well-being. The Greeks turned to the herb when their spirits sagged. Today, herbalists consider borage a diuretic, demulcent, and emollient, and prescribe the plant to treat depression, fevers, bronchitis, and diarrhea. The malic acid and potassium nitrate it contains may be responsible for its diuretic effects. Poultices of leaves may be useful in cooling and soothing skin and reducing inflammation and swelling. The plant also has expectorant properties.

The crisp flavor of borage flowers complements cheese, fish, poultry, most vegetables, salads, iced beverages, pickles, and salad dressings. You can eat small amounts of young leaves: Steam well or sauté as you would spinach so the leaves are no longer prickly.

Pick blossoms as they open and use the flowers in foods or preserve them in vinegar to use later.

BURNET

Useful to control bleeding, burnet's name, in fact, means "to drink up blood." The herb is considered helpful in treating vaginal discharges and diarrhea. Burnet leaves contain vitamin C and tannins; the latter gives it astringent properties. Practitioners of traditional Chinese medicine use the root topically on wounds and burns to reduce inflammation and the risk of infection. It is also used to treat gum disease. While burnet is rarely used medicinally in North America, Europeans and Russians still use it in their folk medicine. It is used to heal ulcerative colitis as a folk remedy in Northern Europe and Russia. Apparently, its medicinal properties are due to more than simply the astringent tannins it contains. Russian research shows that the leaves improve circulation to the uterus, especially in pregnant women. The leaves also have immune-enhancing properties that may help correct some abnormalities during pregnancy.

In the kitchen, use tender, young, well-chopped leaves in salads, vinegars, butters, and iced beverages. Add leaves to vinegars, marinades, and cheese spreads.

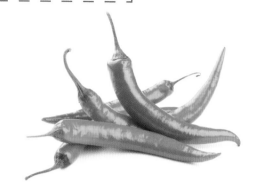

CAYENNE

Cayenne's angular branches and stems may look purplish. Its red podlike fruits are extremely hot. Flowers, which appear in drooping clusters on long stems, are star-shaped and yellowish-white. Leaves are long and elliptical. Cayenne grows naturally in the tropics, but gardeners in most parts of the United States can grow it with success.

Cayenne has many medicinal uses. The main ingredient in cayenne is capsaicin, a powerful stimulant responsible for the pepper's heat. Although it can set your mouth on fire, cayenne, ironically, is good for your digestive system and is now known to help heal ulcers! It reduces substance P, a chemical that carries pain messages from the skin's nerve endings, so it reduces pain when applied topically. A cayenne cream is now in use to treat psoriasis, postsurgical pain, shingles, and nerve damage from diabetes. It may even help you burn off extra pounds. Researchers in England have found that about ¼ ounce of cayenne burns from 45 to 76 calories by increasing metabolism.

Taking cayenne internally stabilizes blood pressure. You can apply powdered, dry cayenne as a poultice over wounds to stop bleeding. And in the kitchen, cayenne spices up any food it touches.

Pick cayenne peppers after the fruits have turned red. Dry immediately and store in a cool, dry place. You can also freeze cayenne peppers or preserve them in oil or vinegar.

Add a pinch of cayenne powder to other herbal infusions to treat colds and influenza. Simmer 3 tablespoons cayenne in 1 cup of cider vinegar. Do not strain. Shake before using. Take 1 teaspoon (4 droppers full) straight or add it to ½ cup warm water or tea for colds, flu, or sore throat.

PRECAUTIONS

Overexposure to the skin can produce pain, dizziness, and a rapid pulse. Alcohol or fat, such as whole milk, neutralizes the reaction. If you touch a pepper and then rub your eyes or nose, you could inflame those sensitive tissues.

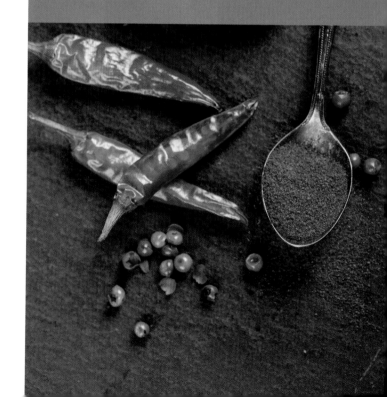

CHIVES

Chives produces tight clumps of long, thin, grasslike leaves that resemble those of onion in appearance and taste. The herb produces abundant, small, rose-purple, globe-shaped flower heads in early summer. Chives may be planted as edging, grown alone, or grown with other plants in containers.

Archaeologists tell us that chives has been in use for at least 5,000 years. By the 16th century, it was a popular European garden herb. Chives' few medicinal properties derive from the sulfur-rich oil found in all members of the onion family. The oil is antiseptic and may help lower blood pressure, but it must be consumed in fairly large quantities. Chives' pleasant taste—like that of mild, sweet onions—complements the flavor of most foods. Use fresh minced leaves in dishes containing potatoes, artichokes, asparagus, cauliflower, corn, tomatoes, peas, carrots, spinach, poultry, fish, veal, cheese, eggs, and, of course, in cream cheese atop your bagel or in sour cream on a baked potato. Add chives at the last minute for best flavor. Flowers are good additions to salads and may be preserved in vinegars.

The best way to derive chives' benefits is to add minced leaves liberally to cooked dishes or use a chive vinegar.

CORIANDER

Coriander's bright green, lacy leaves resemble those of flat-leaved Italian parsley when they first spring up from seed, but they become more fern-like as the plant matures.

Coriander has been cultivated for 3,000 years. The Hebrews, who used coriander seed as one of their Passover herbs, probably learned about it from the ancient Egyptians, who revered the plant. The Romans and Greeks used coriander for medicinal purposes and as a spice and preservative. The Chinese believed coriander could make a human immortal. Throughout northern Europe, people would suck on candy-coated coriander seeds when they had indigestion; chewing the seeds soothes an upset stomach, relieves flatulence, aids digestion, and improves appetite. Poultices of coriander seeds have been used to relieve the pain of rheumatism. The Chinese prescribe the tea to treat dysentery and measles. Coriander relieves inflammation and headaches. But its most popular medicinal use has been to flavor strong-tasting medicines and to prevent intestinal gripping common with some laxative formulas.

Harvest only fresh, young leaves, and freeze them promptly or preserve them in vinegar. Harvest seeds when they start to turn brown. Cut a whole plant and hang-dry upside down inside paper bags to catch seeds.

PRECAUTIONS

Very large doses are narcotic, but it is unlikely you could eat the quantity needed to produce this effect.

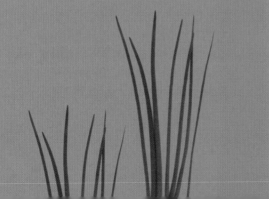

GARLIC

Like its cousin the onion, garlic produces a compound bulb composed of numerous cloves encased in a papery sheath. Flowers are small and white to pinkish. Long, slender green leaves arise from the bulb.

Garlic has been prized for millennia, used by the Egyptians, Hebrews, Romans, Greeks, and Chinese. Garlic is one of the most extensively researched and widely used of plants. Its actions are diverse and affect nearly every body system. The herb boasts antibiotic, antifungal, and antiviral properties and is reported to be effective against many influenza strains, as well as herpes simplex type I. During World War I, field physicians applied garlic juice to infected wounds. Allicin, which gives garlic its distinctive odor, is as effective as a 1 percent penicillin solution in destroying bacteria, fungi, and yeast.

Garlic has been used to treat streptococcal infections, dysentery, whooping cough, and even tuberculosis. Several of garlic's sulfur compounds are noxious to parasites. Garlic inhibits blood clotting and keeps platelets from clumping, which improves blood flow and reduces the risk of stroke. It reduces cholesterol levels, making it a preventive for heart diseases. One study found that people who regularly ate garlic had almost half as many heart attacks. Garlic lowers blood pressure by relaxing vein and artery walls, keeping them open to improve blood flow. Constituents in garlic appear to increase insulin levels and lower high blood sugar levels.

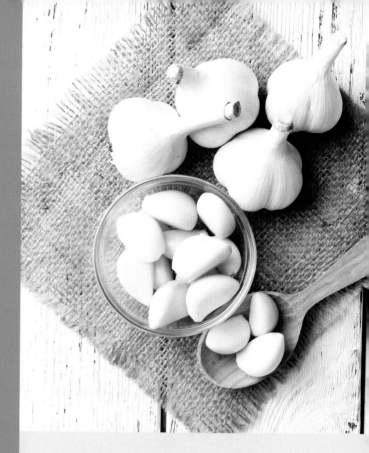

PRECAUTIONS

Some people who consume large amounts of garlic feel nauseous or hot or have gas and bloating. Garlic juice may irritate the skin or mucous membranes of sensitive people.

MEDICINAL USE

One of the best ways to consume garlic is to eat it raw. When cooked, the stronger the flavor is, the more medicinal value it has. You can also take 1 to 2 capsules of garlic two to three times a day. Take ¼ teaspoon (1 dropper full) of garlic tincture in a glass of water, two to four times a day. A good antifungal treatment is to use garlic vinegar (garlic tincture made with vinegar).

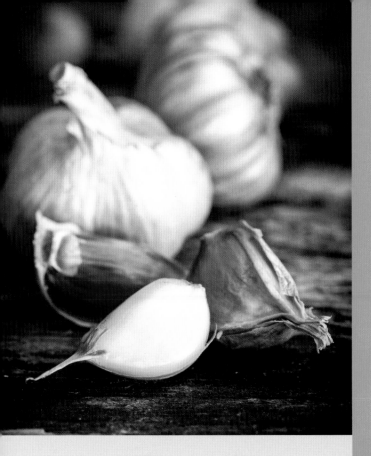

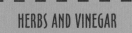
HORSERADISH

Have you ever bitten into a roast beef sandwich and thought your nose was on fire? The sandwich probably contained horseradish. Even a tiny taste of this potent condiment seems to go straight to your nose. Whether on a sandwich or in a herbal preparation, horseradish clears sinuses, increases facial circulation, and promotes expulsion of mucus.

Horseradish is helpful for sinus infections because it encourages your body to get rid of mucus. One way a sinus infection starts is with the accumulation of thick mucus in the sinuses: Stagnant mucus is the perfect breeding ground for bacteria to multiply and cause a painful infection. Horseradish can help thin and move out older, thicker mucus accumulations. If you are prone to developing sinus infections, try taking horseradish the minute you feel a cold coming on. Herbalists also recommend horseradish for common colds, influenza, and lung congestion. Incidentally, don't view the increase of mucus production after horseradish therapy as a sign your cold is worsening. The free-flowing mucus is a positive sign that your body is ridding itself of wastes.

Horseradish has a mild natural antibiotic effect and it stimulates urine production. Thus, it has been used for urinary infections.

Occasionally, horseradish is used topically to alleviate the pain of arthritis and nerve irritation. Horseradish also has been used as a poultice to treat infected wounds.

PICKLED GARLIC

Since vinegar and garlic are both good for you, why not combine the two and make pickled garlic? Simply peel some garlic cloves, cube them, and let them sit for 10 to 15 minutes to form allicin. Then add the garlic to your favorite vinegar.

Vinegar helps garlic form healthful sulfur-containing compounds that are not otherwise formed in large amounts. The longer the garlic is in the vinegar, the more sulfur compounds it forms. Store your pickled garlic in the refrigerator and add it to salads and vegetable side dishes. What a delicious way to take your medicine—maybe a pickled clove a day will keep the doctor away.

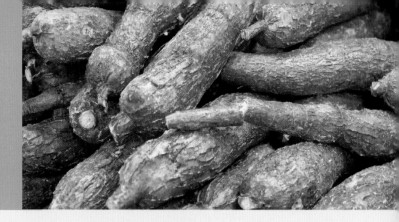

PRECAUTIONS
Avoid prolonged exposure to horseradish's volatile fumes, which may irritate the lungs and cause a burning sensation.

PREPARATION AND USAGE

Horseradish root keeps for several months in a re-sealable plastic bag in the refrigerator. (Fresh root is superior as a medicine, but commercially prepared horseradish will do in a pinch.) Grate the horserad-ish in a food processor or blender. Add honey or sugar and vinegar to taste (about 2 tablespoons honey or sugar and 1 tablespoon vinegar per cup of horseradish).

Tincture: Take ¼ to ½ teaspoon of horseradish tincture at a time, straight or in warm water, every hour or so to clear head congestion.

HORSERADISH-CRANBERRY HOLIDAY RELISH
Blend ingredients in a blender or food processor to create a beautiful pink condiment that will get your taste buds' attention, as well as treat your winter colds.

1	cup freshly grated horseradish root
2	cups organic cranberries
2	Tbsp vinegar
¼	cup honey
½	cup sour cream

LAVENDER
Perhaps the smell of lavender reminds you of soap. That's because lavender is a prime ingredient of many soaps. Its name, in fact, derives from the Latin "to wash." The Romans and Greeks used lavender in the bath. Lavender is also found commercially in shaving creams, colognes, and perfumes. It is used in many cosmetics and aromatherapy products because it is so versa-tile, and its fragrance blends so well with other herbs. Studies show that the scent is very relaxing. Lavender's scent is also a remedy for headache and nervous tension.

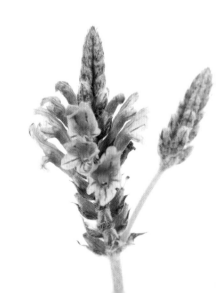

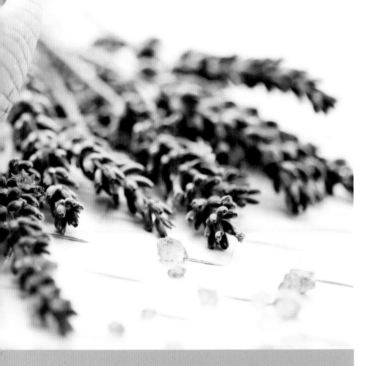

Lavender cosmetics are good for all complexion types. It is an excellent skin healer: It promotes the healing of burns, abrasions, infected sores, and other types of inflammations, including varicose veins. It is also a popular hair rinse. The herb is a carminative and antispasmodic. It is most often used for sore muscles in the form of a massage oil. As recently as World War I, lavender was used in the field as a disinfectant for wounds; herbalists still recommend it for that purpose. Lavender destroys several viruses, including many that cause colds and flu. It also relieves lung and sinus congestion. Lavender flowers may be added to vinegars, jellies, sachets, and potpourri. Place a sprig of lavender in a drawer to freshen linens. And dried flowers make wonderful herbal arrangements, although they are fragile.

MUSTARD

You'll recognize species of the large mustard family by their strong smell and four-petaled flowers. Mustard flowers are small and yellow, and the petals resemble a Maltese cross. Lower leaves are pinnately lobed or coarsely toothed; upper leaves are not as lobed. The plant flowers in early summer. Mustards grow just about everywhere.

Mustard has many medicinal uses. Some of us are old enough to remember getting a mustard plaster when ill with a cold. Mustard seeds warm the skin and open the lungs to make breathing easier. Mustard plasters may also relieve rheumatism, toothache, sore muscles, and arthritis. Its chief constituent, mustard oil, gives it its heat and flavor. These constituents also make mustard an appetite stimulant and a powerful irritant. Mustard in small doses improves digestion. Young leaves are vitamin-rich additions to salads, or they can be boiled with onions and salt pork.

MAKE YOUR OWN!

You haven't really tasted mustard until you've made it yourself. To make mustard from seeds, boil $1/3$ cup cider vinegar, $2/3$ cup cider, 2 tablespoons honey, $1/8$ tablespoon turmeric, and up to 1 teaspoon salt. While hot, combine with $1/4$ cup ground mustard seeds. Blend in a food processor. After the mixture is smooth, add 1 tablespoon olive oil. This recipe makes $1^1/4$ cups of mustard.

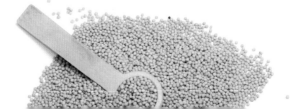

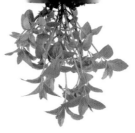

› APPLE CIDER VINEGAR

MARJORAM

Marjoram is a bushy, spreading, fairly hardy perennial that is grown as an annual in freezing climates. It produces small, oval, gray-green, velvety leaves and knotlike shapes that blossom into tiny white or pink flowers from August through September. The herb makes an attractive potted plant that may be brought inside when temperatures fall.

The Greeks knew marjoram as "joy of the mountains" and used it as a remedy for sadness. Herbalists have prescribed marjoram to treat asthma, increase sweating, lower fevers, encourage menstruation, and, especially, relieve indigestion. European singers preserved their voices with marjoram tea sweetened with honey. The herb has antioxidant and antifungal properties. Recent studies show marjoram inhibits several viruses, including the herpesvirus. Marjoram gargles and steam treatments relieve sinus congestion and hay fever. A massage oil made from marjoram helps relieve muscle and menstrual cramps. The diluted essential oil can be rubbed into sore gums, in place of clove oil. Aromatherapists use the scent to relax the mind, induce sleep, and even relieve grief.

Marjoram tastes like a mild oregano with a hint of balsam. Add leaves to salads, beef, veal, lamb, roasted poultry, fish, patés, and vegetables such as carrots, cauliflower, eggplant, mushrooms, parsnips, potatoes, squash, and tomatoes. The herb also complements stews, sautés, marinades, dressings, butters, oils, vinegars, and cheese spreads. Its antioxidant properties are so potent they have been shown to be excellent food preservatives.

NASTURTIUM

Description: Nasturtiums produce distinctive, blue-green circular leaves on fleshy stems. The plants come in a variety of types, ranging from compact bushes to spreading vines. They produce large, attractive blooms that range from pale yellow, pink, and apricot to deep, rich gold, orange, and burgundy.

Spanish conquerors brought nasturtiums from Peru to Spain. Soon these lovely flowering herbs spread across the continent. Nasturtium leaves have a peppery flavor, make good additions to salads, and can be added to sandwiches. Flower buds may be cured in vinegar and used like capers. Pull off the individual petals to add color and flavor to a salad. The natural antibiotic in nasturtiums is effective even against some microorganisms that have built up a resistance to antibiotic drugs. The leaves and flowers fight infections of the lung and reproductive and urinary tracts.

Harvest fresh leaves and flowers as needed. Pickle unripe seeds in vinegar and use them in salads.

Nasturtiums are medicinal when eaten. You can use them as a tincture; however, they are seldom used in this form. Sometimes the leaves are added to herb teas. One tasty way to use nasturtium is to make an herbal vinegar to use on salads.

PRECAUTIONS

Large amounts of the seeds act as a strong laxative (purgative).

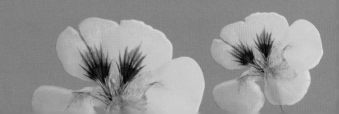

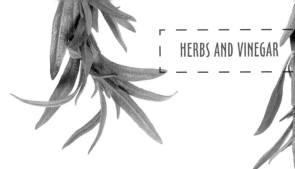

RASPBERRY

Native to North America and Europe, this shrubby, thorny plant, also known as hindberry and bramble, quickly spread around the world. You'll find raspberry thickets along the edges of woods and in untended fields. The raspberry plant produces a prickly stem. Its flowers are white and appear in the spring and summer of its second year. Berries ripen in June and July. Each fruit is composed of lots of little fruits, or drupelets, which give it its familiar shape. The plant produces erect shoots or canes that, in time, flop over and reproduce.

Long revered for its healing properties, raspberry is an astringent, stimulant, and tonic. Seventeenth-century English herbalist Nicholas Culpepper recommended raspberry for a number of ailments, including "fevers, ulcers, putrid sores of the mouth and secret parts... spitting blood...piles...stones of the kidney... and too much flowing of women's courses." American Indians used raspberry as a treatment for wounds. And contemporary herbalists prescribe raspberry for diarrhea, nausea, vomiting, and morning sickness. In addition, raspberry leaves are thought to tone uterine muscles and, thus, have long been used by pregnant women to prevent miscarriage and reduce labor pains. They can be used throughout pregnancy. They relieve menstrual cramps if taken as a tonic over a period of time. Raspberry leaves are also good for women with uterine problems such as fibroids, endometriosis, or excessive menstrual bleeding.

Freeze or preserve the fruit in vinegar.

SAVORY

This attractive annual has soft, flat, gray-green, narrow leaves. The plant has a light, airy appearance. Winter savory is a hardy perennial. Summer savory is tastier but has a shorter growing season than winter savory: It flowers from midsummer to the first frost.

The Romans believed savory was sacred to satyrs, mythical man-goats who were said to roam the forests. The Romans also planted it near beehives to increase honey production. They used savory to flavor vinegars and introduced the herb to England, where the Saxons adopted and named it for its spicy taste. Winter savory was said to curb sexual appetite; summer savory, to increase it. Guess which variety was most popular? Summer savory has antiseptic and astringent properties, so it has been used to treat diarrhea and mild sore throats. Like many culinary herbs, it aids digestion, stimulates appetite, and relieves a minor upset stomach and eliminates gas—probably one reason it is so popular to flavor bean dishes. It also kills several types of intestinal worms.

In the kitchen, summer savory's flavor, reminiscent of thyme, brings out the best in butters, vinegars, beans, soups, eggs, peas, eggplant, asparagus, onions, and cabbage. It is one of the flavorings in salami and other commercial foods. It is often considered a lighter substitute for sage or thyme.

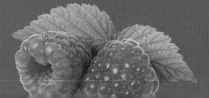

TARRAGON

This perennial has long, narrow, pointed leaves, but its flowers rarely appear. Be sure to get the French rather than the Russian variety of tarragon. The Russian variety looks much the same but has somewhat narrower, lighter green leaves, and it flowers and produces seed. But Russian tarragon has less of the sweetly aromatic flavor of its French cousin.

Thomas Jefferson was one of the first Americans to grow this lovely and useful plant. Tarragon stimulates appetite, relieves gas and colic, and makes a good local anesthetic for toothaches. Tarragon has antifungal and antioxidant properties and has been used to preserve foods. It's also found in perfumes, soaps, cosmetics, condiments, and liqueurs. One of the French fines herbes, tarragon has a strong flavor that may overpower foods, so use it sparingly in salads and sauces, including remoulade, tartar, and bearnaise sauces. Tarragon enhances fish, pork, beef, lamb, game, poultry, patés, rice, barley, vinegars, mayonnaise, and butter. It also goes well with a number of vegetables, including potatoes, tomatoes, carrots, onions, beets, asparagus, mushrooms, cauliflower, and broccoli.

Pick leaves or 3- to 4-inch growth tips at any time for fresh use. Cut the stems and hang to dry. Don't dry tarragon too long or it will lose its flavor. Store immediately in an airtight container. You can also capture tarragon's flavor in vinegar.

THYME

These tiny-leaved, wide-spreading perennials make a good inexpensive ground cover that can be clipped and mowed regularly. Thyme's profuse lilac to pink blooms appear in June and July and are especially attractive to bees.

You may have noticed thyme's distinctive flavor in cough medicines. Thymol, a prime constituent, is found in a number of them. Thymol is also used commercially to make colognes, aftershaves, lotions, soaps, detergents, and cosmetics. Thyme also was used as an antiseptic to treat wounds as recently as World War I. In fact, it is one of the most potent antiseptics of all the herbs. Thymol is found in many mouthwashes and gargles for sore throats and mouth and gum infections. It is one of the main ingredients in Listerine, along with compounds from eucalyptus and peppermint. This commercial mouthwash was found to cause 34 percent less gum inflammation than other brands and decrease plaque formation on the teeth. Vapor balms, used to rub on the chest to relieve congestion, also contain thymol. Thyme destroys fungal infections. Its antispasmodic qualities make it useful for treating asthma, whooping cough, stomach cramps, gas, colic, and headache. It also reduces compounds in the body that produce menstrual cramps. Thyme preparations increase circulation in the area where applied.

One of the French fines herbes, thyme complements salads, veal, lamb, beef, poultry, fish, stuffing, patés, sausage, stews, soups, bread, butters, mayonnaise, vinegars, mustard, eggs, cheese, and many vegetables, including tomatoes, onions, eggplant, leeks, mushrooms, asparagus, and green beans.

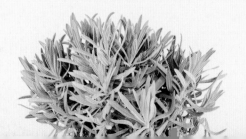

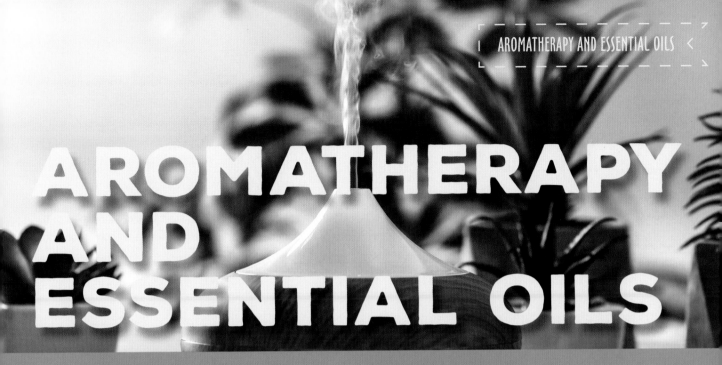

AROMATHERAPY AND ESSENTIAL OILS

Apple cider vinegar is useful on its own—but it can be an even more powerful force when combined with other healing elements. The old saying claims that "oil and vinegar don't mix," but vinegar can be paired with the essential oils used in aromatherapy. Essential oils are generally mixed with another sub-stance, called a carrier oil. While vegetable oil and alcohol are more commonly used as carrier oils, vinegar has its place as a carrier oil in the practice of aromatherapy. In this section we'll look at some of the basics of aromatherapy, certain essential oils that pair well with vinegar as a carrier oil, and some common health conditions and aromatherapy recipes for treating those conditons.

WHAT IS AROMATHERAPY?

The burning of fragrant woods, leaves, needles, and tree gums as incense is thought to be the earliest form of aromatherapy. This practice probably arose from the discovery that some firewoods, such as cypress and cedar, filled the air with scent when they burned. In fact, our modern word perfume is derived from the Latin *per fumum,* which means "through smoke."

As civilization became more advanced, incense, body oils, and aromatic waters were combined into blends to heal the mind, body, and spirit. Thus, throughout the world, aroma became an integral part of healing and lay the foundation for our use of aromatherapy today.

Remember the heady fragrance of an herb or flower garden on a hot summer's day, or the crisp smell of an orange as you peel it? These odors are the fragrance of the plant's essential oils, the potent, volatile, and aromatic substance contained in various parts of the plant, including its flowers, leaves, roots, wood, seeds, fruit, and bark. The essential oils carry concentrations of the plant's healing properties—those same proper-ties that traditional Western medicine utilizes in many drugs.

Aromatherapy simply means the application of those healing powers—it is a fragrant cure. Professional aromatherapists focus very specifically on the controlled use of essential oils to treat ailments and disease and to promote physical and emotional well-being.

Aromatherapy doesn't just work through the sense of smell alone, however. Inhalation is only one application method. Essential oils can also be applied to the skin. When used topically, the oils penetrate the skin, taking direct action on body tissues and organs in the vicinity of application. They also enter the bloodstream and are carried throughout the body. Of course, when applied topically the fragrance of the essential oil is also inhaled.

There are three different modes of action in the body: pharmacological, which affects the chemistry of the body; physiological, which affects the ability of the body to function and process; and psychological, which affects emotions and attitudes. These three modes interact continuously. Aromatherapy is so powerful partly because it affects all three modes. You choose the application method based on where you most want the effects concentrated and on what is most convenient and pleasing to you.

Aromatherapy is actually an aspect of a larger category of healing treatment known as herbal medicine. Herbal medicine also utilizes the healing powers of plants to treat physical and emotional problems, but it uses the whole plant or parts of the plant, such as leaves, flowers, roots, and seeds, rather than the essential oil. Aromatherapy and herbal medicine can be used individually, or they can be used jointly to augment potential healing benefits.

THERAPEUTIC USES OF ESSENTIAL OILS

You can treat a wide range of physical problems with aromatherapy. Almost all essential oils have antiseptic properties and are able to fight infection and destroy bacteria, fungi, yeast, parasites, and/or viruses. Many essential oils also reduce aches and pain, soothe or rout inflammations and spasms, stimulate the immune system and insulin and hormone production, affect blood circulation, dissolve mucus and open nasal passages, or aid digestion—just to mention a few of their amazing properties.

Aromatherapy can also have a considerable influence on our emotions. Sniffing clary sage, for example, can quell panic, while the fragrance released by peeling an orange can make you feel more optimistic. Since your mind strongly influences your health and is itself a powerful healing tool, it makes aromatherapy's potential even more exciting.

Many essential oils perform more than one function, so having just a half-dozen or so on hand will help you treat a wide range of common physical ailments and emotional problems. The beauty of aromatherapy is that you can create a blend of oils that will benefit both in one treatment. For example, you can blend a combination of essential oils that not only stops indigestion, but also reduces the nervous condition that encouraged it. Or, you could design an aromatherapy body lotion that both improves your complexion and relieves depression.

HOW DO ESSENTIAL OILS WORK?

Plants take the light of the sun, the minerals of the earth, and the carbon dioxide exhaled by humans and animals and, through photosynthesis, transform them into the building blocks of medicine. Among the most important therapeutic compounds manufactured by plants are essential oils. These volatile oils contain a variety of active constituents and are also responsible for each plant's unique fragrance.

The basic elements of carbon, hydrogen, and oxygen combine to form the different organic molecular compounds that produce aromas. So far, more than 30,000 of these molecular compounds have been identified and named. Most individual essential oils consist of many different aromatic molecular compounds. In fact, the essential oil from just one plant may contain as many as one hundred different fragrance molecules. In nature there are thousands of plants, all with unique fragrances that are comprised of different combinations of these molecules.

Each molecular compound has characteristic scents and actions on the body. Some may be cooling and relaxing, while others are warming and stimulating. Some are better for treating indigestion, while others are antiseptic.

Essential oil molecules enter the body through the nose and the skin. Since these molecules are extremely small and float easily through the air, you can simply inhale them into your lungs, which then disperse them into your bloodstream. The blood quickly carries them throughout your body. Essential oil molecules are also small enough to be absorbed through the pores of the skin. Once absorbed, some molecules enter the bloodstream, while others remain in the area of application or evaporate into the air. How much goes where depends on the size of the essential oil molecules, the method of application (massage increases absorption), and the carrier containing the essential oil, be it vinegar, alcohol, vegetable oil, or water. This makes essential oils perfect for healing a specific skin problem as well as the entire body.

BUYING ESSENTIAL OILS

Shopping for essential oils can be confusing. How can you, as a consumer, make educated decisions on what to buy? A few tricks of the trade should help you sniff your way through all the confusion.

• Buy from companies that have established a reputation for quality.

• When buying from an unknown company, purchase only one or two of their oils in small amounts (a quarter ounce, dram, or even less), even though it will cost proportionately more than a larger quantity.

• Put one drop of the essential oil on a piece of paper. Most oils are so volatile they will evaporate quickly, leaving no oily mark. The presence of an oil mark indicates that it's been adulterated. A few highly pigmented oils such as the deep blue German chamomile or brown patchouli will leave color stains, but they will not look or feel oily.

• If you are lucky enough to sniff and compare many oils, you will quickly develop a scent overload. Breathe several times through a scarf or cap of pure wool to clear your smell receptors.

• Check for scents that are fuller, rounder, and more complex. A little goes a long way, so you will need to use less in your products.

STORAGE

Once you've purchased quality essential oils, you certainly will want to keep them that way. Store them in glass containers. Some essential oils can actually dissolve plastic, and storing them even temporarily in it may contaminate the oil. Don't store essential oils in dropper bottles either, as it doesn't take long for the rubber seals and squeeze bulbs to melt into a gooey mess.

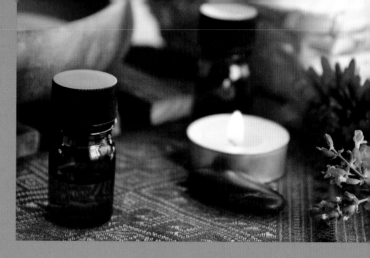

The color of the bottle doesn't really matter. Just be sure to keep all essential oils out of direct sunlight and away from heat so they don't lose their potency.

Essential oils are natural preservatives and will help preserve your carrier oils. Their scent will change and fade over time, however, and eventually lose its quality. Properly stored, most oils will keep for at least several years. The citrus oils, such as orange and lemon, are most vulnerable to losing their smell, but even they will keep for a couple of years if refrigerated.

A few essential oils, including patchouli, clary sage, benzoin, vetiver, and sandalwood, actually help fix the scent of other aromas combined with them. And they get better with age. The same is true for thick resins such as myrrh. Patchouli that has been stored for many years smells so rich, few people recognize it— even those who otherwise dislike it! Essential oils such as these become yet more valuable with age.

Making aromatherapy products to use for healing or as skin care products is as easy as it is fun. And you don't need much in the way of equipment to get started. In fact, you probably have most of what you need in your kitchen already. Add some bottles, some essential oils, and some carrier oils to your supplies and you'll be ready to begin experimenting.

CARRIERS

Mixing your essential oil with a carrier is the most popular way of preparing aromatherapy products. It is also the easiest way to dilute essential oils in preparation for use. There are several choices of carriers; the most common are vegetable oil, alcohol, water, and vinegar. The carrier you choose will depend on how you plan to apply your treatment. For a massage or body oil, vegetable oil is the best choice. For a liniment, you may prefer alcohol as your base because it doesn't leave an oily residue. A room spray only needs a water base, while aloe vera juice is perfect for a complexion spray.

Some aromatherapy preparations incorporate vinegar. It is actually a better base for both skin and hair than alcohol, but some people are put off by its initial smell. The smell dissipates rather quickly, however, and you'll be pleased with the result if you try it. Vinegar is antiseptic, although not as antiseptic as alcohol. Its acidity helps restore the acid mantle or pH-balance to the skin and hair. For this purpose, apple cider vinegar is best, although many people prefer white vinegar because it has no color. Vinegar is water soluble, so you can dilute it with distilled water if you find its smell or sting too strong for the product you are making. Distilled water is used because it doesn't contain chlorine or other city water additives and has none of the bacteria found in well water.

When preparing recipes to be used by the elderly, the very young (less than 12 years of age), or anyone who is very ill or frail, be sure to cut the amount of essential oils in half, keeping the carrier (vegetable oil, water, alcohol, vinegar, etc.) the same. These people are so sensitive that they will react equally well to the smaller amount.

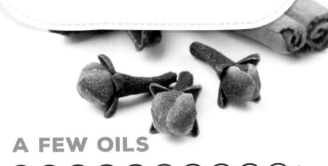

A FEW OILS

CLOVE

In ancient China, courtiers at the Han court held cloves in their mouths to freshen their breath before they had an audience with the emperor. Today, cloves are still used to sweeten breath. Modern dental preparations numb tooth and gum pain and quell infection with clove essential oil or its main constituent, eugenol. Simply inhaling the fragrance was once said to improve eyesight and fend off the plague. Clove's scent developed a reputation, now backed by science, for being stimulating. The fragrance was also believed to be an aphrodisiac. Cloves were so valuable that a Frenchman risked his life to steal a clove tree from the Dutch colonies in Indonesia and plant it in French ground. Once established, the slender evergreen trees bear buds for at least a century. The familiar clove buds used to poke hams and flavor mulled wine are picked while still unripe and dried before being shipped or distilled into essential oil.

PRINCIPAL CONSTITUENTS: Eugenol, eugenyl acetate, caryophyllene

SCENT: The fragrance is powerful, sweet-spicy, and hot, with fruity top notes.

THERAPEUTIC PROPERTIES: Antibacterial, antifungal, antihistamine; decreases gas and indigestion, clears mucous from the lungs, expels intestinal worms

USED FOR: As an antiseptic and pain-reliever, clove essential oil relieves toothaches, flu, colds, and bronchial congestion.

In a heating liniment, clove essential oil helps sore muscles and arthritis. Liniments increase circulation. Rub them externally on the skin to warm muscles and to reduce muscle and joint pain. Fitness experts suggest applying liniment before exercising, not afterwards, so that it can work like a mini-warm-up, heating muscles so they will stretch better. (Don't use this as an excuse to skimp on your stretches, however!) Make a quick and easy liniment by adding 15–20 drops of clove for every ounce of vinegar. The same proportion will work if you substitute cinnamon or peppermint for clove.

Mix 30 drops of clove essential oil in one ounce of apple cider vinegar, shake well, and dab on athlete's foot.

WARNINGS: The essential oil irritates skin and mucous membranes, so be sure to dilute it before use. Clove leaf is almost pure eugenol; do not use it in aromatherapy preparations.

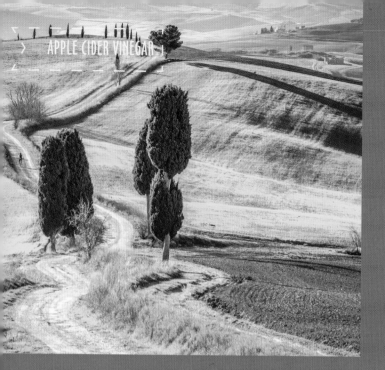

CYPRESS

The landscapes of southern France and Greece are graced with this statuesque evergreen, which first came from the island of Cyprus where it was worshiped as a representation of the goddess Beruth. The tree appears in art and literature as an emblem of generation, death, the immortal soul, and woe. This long association with mortality continues today, for modern Egyptians use cypress wood for coffins, while the French and Americans plant it in graveyards. Greeks say that cypress clears the mind during stressful times and comforts mourners. Cypress stanches bleeding (Hippocrates recommended it for hemorrhoids) and the Chinese chewed its small cones, rich in essential oils and astringents, to heal bleeding gums. The Chinese also revered cypress, but associated it with contemplation because its roots grow in the form of a seated man. The greenish essential oil is distilled from the tree's needles or twigs and sometimes from its cones.

PRINCIPAL CONSTITUENTS: Pinene, camphene, sylvestrene, cymene, sabinol

SCENT: It has a smoky, pungent, pinelike, and spicy scent.

THERAPEUTIC PROPERTIES: Antiseptic, astringent, deodorant; relieves rheumatic pain, relaxes muscle spasms and cramping, stops bleeding, and constricts blood vessels.

USED FOR: Cypress's specialty is treating circulation problems, such as low blood pressure, poor circulation, varicose veins, and hemorrhoids. Because it helps heal broken capillaries and also discourages fluid retention, it is a favored essential oil at menopause. For these uses, add 8 drops to every ounce of cream or lotion and apply gently to the afflicted region a couple of times a day. You can also alleviate laryngitis, spasmodic coughing, and lung congestion just by putting a drop on your pillow. A European folk remedy is to inhale smoke from the burning gum resin to relieve sinus congestion, although inhaling a few drops of the essential oil in steam is a healthier approach. Place a cypress compress over the abdomen to quell excessive menstruation, urinary infection, or inflammation. Because of its astringent, antiseptic, and deodorant properties, dilute about 6 drops of cypress essential oil in vinegar for an oily complexion or to reduce excessive sweating.

EUCALYPTUS

Australia's "blue forests" are named for the haze produced by the tree's essential oil. When you walk through the groves, the blue mist that mutes the surrounding scenery can be almost intoxicating. One can't help but take deep breaths of its refreshing scent—which is perhaps why aromatherapists use it to "clear the air," helping to resolve disagreements in interpersonal conflicts.

Eucalyptus or "gum" trees originated in Australia and Tasmania, but they are now found in subtropical regions all over the globe. They are one of the tallest and fastest growing trees. The eucalyptus tree was introduced at the Paris Exposition in 1867 after the director of the botanical gardens in Melbourne, Australia, suggested that the essential oil might be an antiseptic replacement for cajeput oil. He was right. The French government then planted the fast-growing trees in Algeria to ward off the "noxious gases" thought to be responsible for malaria. It worked, but ironically this was not due to the essential oil, but because the water-hungry trees transformed the marsh into dry land, eliminating the mosquitos' habitat.

Eucalyptus' thick, long, bluish-green leaves are distilled to provide essential oil. Blue gum eucalyptus, the most widely cultivated variety, provides most of the commercially available oil, although with more than 600 species, there are a variety of scents.

A very inexpensive oil, eucalyptus is used liberally to scent aftershaves and colognes and as an antiseptic in mouthwashes and household cleansers.

PRINCIPAL CONSTITUENTS: Cineol or eucalyptol, pinene, limonene, and at least 250 other compounds. Varieties can include citronellal, cineole, cryptone, piperitone.

SCENT: The odor is pungent, sharp, and somewhat camphoraceous.

THERAPEUTIC PROPERTIES: Antibacterial, antiviral, deodorant; clears mucous from the lungs; as a liniment, relieves rheumatic, arthritic, and other types of pain

USED FOR: Highly antiseptic, eucalyptus has long been a household remedy in Australia for

treating everything from flu, fever, and sore throat to skin and muscle pain. Most liniments and vapor rubs contain it or eucalyptol, one of its principal constituents. It is the most popular essential oil steam for relieving sinus and lung congestion such as asthma.

Especially appropriate for skin eruptions and oily complexions, it is also used for acne, herpes, and chicken pox. For a homemade preparation, mix eucalyptus essential oil with an equal amount of apple cider vinegar and dab on problem areas. This mix can also be used as an antiseptic on wounds, boils, and insect bites.

WARNINGS: Do not use during an asthma attack.

LEMONGRASS

What gives Ivory Soap its familiar scent? The not-so-familiar lemongrass. A fast-growing, tall perennial grass originally from India and Sri Lanka, lemongrass found its way into traditional cuisines throughout Southeast Asia. It is used extensively in Thai fish soups and curries and is seen more and more frequently in supermarkets in North America.

An important medicinal and culinary herb in South and Central America, South East Asia, and the Caribbean, it is widely known as "fever grass." India's Ayurvedic medical tradition, for instance, has long used it to treat cholera and

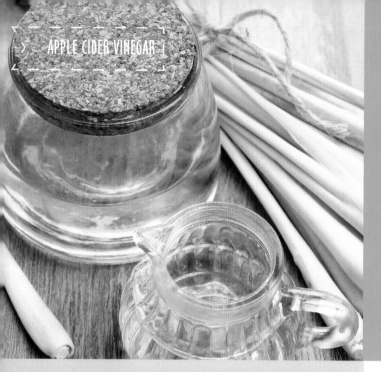

treats pain arising from indigestion, rheumatism, and nerve conditions. Researchers also found this refreshing fragrance to reduce headaches and irritability and to prevent drowsiness.

When added to a hair conditioner, facial water, or vinegar, it counters oily hair and acne by decreasing oil production. Add 12 drops of the essential oil per ounce of apple cider vinegar and dab or spray on the afflicted area. You can spray this same solution in the air, on a counter top, or along walls and floors to discourage insect invasions and mold. Add it to pet shampoos as a bug repellent.

WARNINGS: It is nontoxic, but causes skin sensitivity in some

fevers. A relatively inexpensive essential oil, it's often the source of the lemon scent found in cosmetics and hair preparations. Its pleasant, clean fragrance is also incorporated into soaps, perfumes, and deodorants, and it flavors many canned and frozen foods. No wonder it is one of the ten best-selling essential oils in the world.

PRINCIPAL CONSTITUENTS: Citral (up to 85 percent), myrcene, citronellol, dipentene, farnesol, furfurol, geraniol, and many more

SCENT: The scent is lemon/herbal, grassy, and slightly bitter.

THERAPEUTIC PROPERTIES: Antiseptic, deodorant, astringent; relieves rheumatic and other pain, relaxes nerves

USED FOR: In traditional medicine, lemongrass is usually given in the form of a tea or foot bath made from the fresh herb, from which the patient additionally benefits by inhaling the scent. Lemongrass also

CONDITIONS

BURNS AND SUNBURN

The first step in treating any minor burn or sunburn is to quickly immerse the afflicted area in cold water (about 50°F) containing a few drops of essential oil. Or you can apply a cold compress that has been soaked in the same water. If the person feels overheated or if the eyelids are sunburned, place the compress on the forehead.

Burned skin is tender to the touch, so spraying a remedy is preferable to dabbing it on. A spray also is extra cooling and is especially handy when sunburn covers a large area.

For your burn wash, compress, or spray, lavender is an all-time favorite among aromatherapists. Lavender and aloe vera juice both promote new cell growth, reduce inflammation, stop infection, and decrease pain. Aloe has even been used successfully on radiation burns. There are several other essential oils that reduce the pain of burns and help them heal, so feel free to experiment. Use them in the same proportions suggested for lavender, except rose oil for which 1 drop equals 5 drops of other essential oils.

A small amount of vinegar helps to heal a minor burn and provides an additional cooling effect, but it is painful on an open wound. Reserve it for cases in which the skin is unbroken. In general, stick to treating minor, first-degree burns at home, and leave the care of deeper or more extensive burns to a doctor.

Essential oils for burns and sunburn: chamomile, geranium, lavender, marjoram, peppermint (cooling in small amounts), rose, tea tree

SUNBURN SOOTHER REMEDY

20 drops lavender oil

4 ounces aloe vera juice

200 IU vitamin E oil

1 tablespoon vinegar

Combine ingredients. Shake well before using. Keep this remedy in a spritzer bottle, and use as often as needed. If you keep the spray in the refrigerator, the coolness will provide extra relief. For the best healing, make sure you use aloe vera juice and not drugstore gel. Apply as often as possible until you are healed.

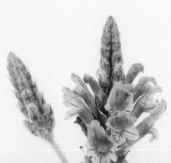

FUNGAL INFECTION/ ATHLETE'S FOOT

Many different fungal infections appear on the skin, and the following treatments can often wipe them out. Most people are familiar with ringworm, especially athlete's foot because it is so common. Athlete's foot is so common because feet sweat and then are cloistered in socks and shoes. This creates the moist environment that fungi really love. If sweating feet are part of the problem, you can use sage to decrease perspiration. Peppermint will help relieve the itching that accompanies a fungal infection. Incorporating the essential oils into a cornstarch powder or a vinegar-based preparation will discourage fungal growth because both are quite drying. Vinegar has the extra benefit of destroying fungal infections.

Some of the most effective antifungal essential oils are tea tree and eucalyptus; lemon eucalyptus is particularly helpful. Lavender, myrrh, and

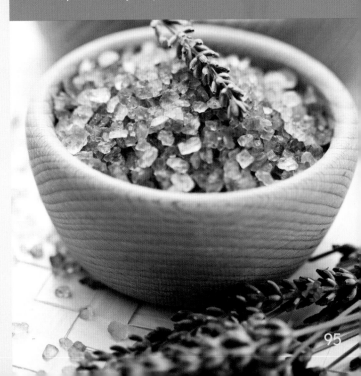

geranium are close seconds. A small amount of peppermint essential oil relieves the itching, and since it stimulates blood circulation, it helps perk you up after a long day on your feet. Don't hesitate to use the same essential oils to treat funguses that creep under nails or affect other parts of the body.

An aromatic foot bath is a great way to treat fungal conditions like athlete's foot or to simply revitalize feet after a long day. You simply can't ask for a better way to take your medicine! If you think you don't have time for such a luxury, why not haul the basin in front of the TV, or read the newspaper or a book while enjoying your soak. Get yourself a basin large enough to accommodate both feet, fill it with warm water, and add several drops of essential oil. Add Epsom salts to relax tight muscles and soreness.

For a complete anti-fungal treatment, start off with a foot bath, hand soak, or wash that covers the afflicted area. Afterward, dry off thoroughly, then apply the Fungal Fighter Solution with vinegar followed by the Fungal Fighter Powder. Do the entire routine at least once a day, and apply either the vinegar or the powder a few extra times.

Essential oils for fungal infection: benzoin, clove, eucalyptus (especially lemon eucalyptus), geranium, lavender, lemongrass, myrrh, peppermint, sandalwood, tea tree, thyme

FUNGAL FIGHTER SOLUTION

12 drops tea tree oil

8 drops geranium oil

3 drops thyme oil

2 drops myrrh oil (expensive, so optional)

1 tablespoon tincture of benzoin

2 ounces apple cider vinegar

Combine the ingredients, and shake well before each use. Dab this solution on the afflicted area, or use it as a wash at least once a day—more often if possible. You can purchase tincture of benzoin at any drugstore.

FUNGAL FIGHTER POWDER

14 drops lemon eucalyptus or tea tree oil

8 drops geranium oil

5 drops sage oil

1 drop peppermint oil

¼ cup cornstarch

Place the cornstarch in a resealable plastic bag. Sprinkle in the essential oils slowly, trying to distribute them evenly through the powder. Close the bag and toss the powder, breaking up any clumps that form. For long-term storage, keep the powder in a sealed plastic bag or glass or ceramic container, although you probably will find a shake bottle with a perforated lid more convenient to dispense it. A variety of these are sold in housewares departments for the kitchen. Use at least once a day, more often if possible.

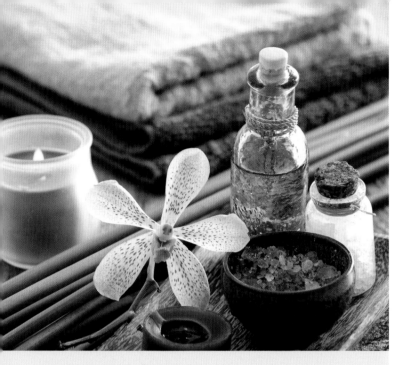

POISON OAK/IVY/ SUMAC REMEDY

- 3   drops lavender oil
- 3   drops cypress oil
- 3   drops peppermint oil
- ½   teaspoon salt
- 1   tablespoon warm water
- 1   tablespoon apple cider vinegar
- 1   ounce calendula tincture

Dissolve the salt in the water and vinegar; then add the other ingredients. Shake well to disperse and again before each use. Apply externally as needed to the rash.

POISON OAK/IVY/SUMAC

The infamous, extremely itchy rash that is caused by touching poison oak or poison ivy is a type of dermatitis that calls for special aromatherapy care. Use a vinegar base, as oil-based products aren't usually recommended in the first stages. However, some people find that a lotion relieves the later dry stage.

Choose essential oils that slow the inflammation and ease the itching. Peppermint may seem an unlikely essential oil to use, but the menthol it contains relieves the painful burning and itching that accompany the rash.

If you can, first soak the affected area in a tepid oatmeal bath. Then apply the remedy described below. Some people find that even warm water is irritating, so experiment with water temperature to find what works best for you.

Essential oils for poison oak/ivy/sumac: chamomile, cypress, geranium, lavender, peppermint

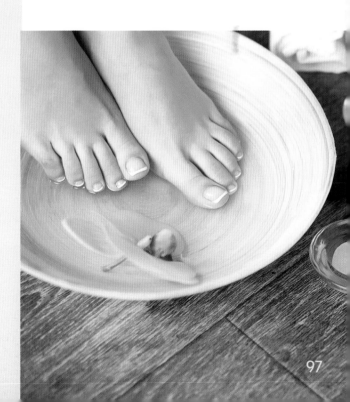

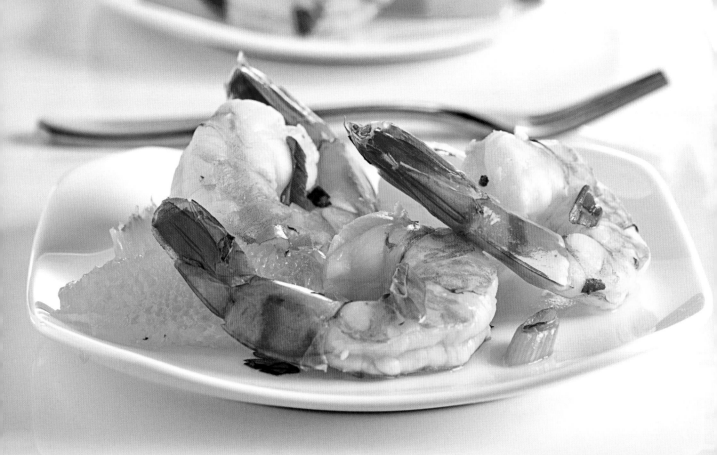

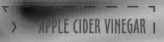
AMAZING APPETIZERS

MARINATED CITRUS SHRIMP
Makes 16 servings

1   pound (about 32) large cooked shrimp peeled and deveined (with tails on)

2   oranges, peeled and cut into segments

1   can (5½ ounces) pineapple chunks in juice, drained and ¼ cup juice reserved

2   green onions, sliced

½   cup orange juice

2   tablespoons lime juice

2   tablespoons apple cider vinegar

2   tablespoons minced fresh cilantro

1   tablespoon olive or vegetable oil

1   clove garlic, minced

½   teaspoon dried basil

½   teaspoon dried tarragon

    White pepper (optional)

1. Combine shrimp, orange segments, pineapple chunks and green onions in large resealable food storage bag. Mix orange juice, reserved pineapple juice, lime juice, vinegar, cilantro, oil, garlic, basil and tarragon in medium bowl; pour over shrimp mixture, turning to coat. Season with white pepper, if desired.

2. Marinate in refrigerator 2 hours or up to 8 hours before serving.

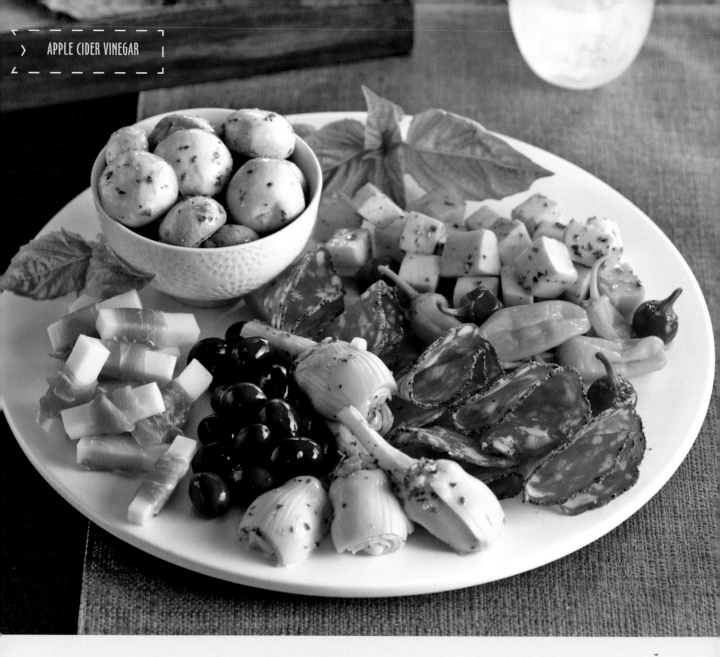

MARINATED MUSHROOMS

3	tablespoons lemon juice	½	teaspoon salt	½	cup extra virgin olive oil
2	tablespoons chopped fresh parsley	¼	teaspoon dried tarragon	½	pound small or medium fresh mushrooms, stems removed
1	clove garlic, crushed	⅛	teaspoon black pepper		

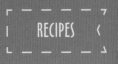
ANTIPASTO WITH MARINATED MUSHROOMS
Makes 6 to 8 servings

Marinated Mushrooms (recipe below)

4   teaspoons red wine vinegar

½   teaspoon dried basil

½   teaspoon dried oregano

Black pepper

¼   cup extra virgin olive oil

4   ounces mozzarella cheese, cut into ½-inch cubes

4   ounces prosciutto or cooked ham, thinly sliced

4   ounces provolone cheese, cut into 2-inch sticks

1   jar (10 ounces) pepperoncini peppers, drained

8   ounces hard salami, thinly sliced

2   jars (6 ounces each) marinated artichoke hearts, drained

6   ounces black olives

Fresh basil leaves or chives (optional)

1. Prepare Marinated Mushrooms; set aside. Combine vinegar, dried basil, oregano and black pepper in small bowl. Add oil; whisk until well blended. Add mozzarella; stir to coat. Marinate, covered, in refrigerator at least 2 hours.

2. Drain mozzarella, reserving marinade. Wrap 1 prosciutto slice around each provolone stick; roll up remaining slices separately.

3. Arrange mozzarella, prosciutto-wrapped provolone sticks, prosciutto rolls, Marinated Mushrooms, pepperoncini, salami, artichoke hearts and olives on large platter. Drizzle reserved marinade over pepperoncini, artichoke hearts and olives. Garnish with fresh basil. Serve with small forks or toothpicks.

1. Combine lemon juice, parsley, garlic, salt, tarragon and pepper in medium bowl. Add oil; whisk until well blended. Add mushrooms; stir to coat. Marinate, covered, in refrigerator 4 hours or overnight, stirring occasionally.

2. Drain mushrooms; reserve marinade for dressing.

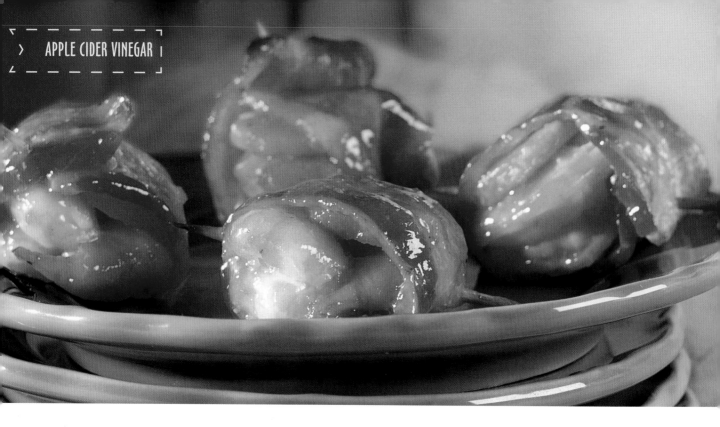

APRICOT BBQ GLAZED SHRIMP AND BACON
Makes 36 appetizers

1   can (8 ounces) sliced water chestnuts, drained

36 medium raw shrimp, peeled and deveined (about 1¼ pounds)

9   slices bacon, each cut into 4 pieces

⅓   cup apricot fruit spread

⅓   cup barbecue sauce

1   tablespoon grated fresh ginger

1   tablespoon apple cider vinegar

⅛   teaspoon red pepper flakes

1. Preheat broiler. Place 1 water chestnut slice on top of each shrimp. Wrap 1 piece of bacon around shrimp and water chestnut; secure with toothpick. Repeat with remaining water chestnuts, shrimp and bacon.

2. Line broiler pan with foil; insert broiler rack. Coat broiler rack with nonstick cooking spray. Place shrimp on rack.

3. Combine fruit spread, barbecue sauce, ginger, vinegar and red pepper flakes in small bowl; stir to blend. Brush sauce evenly over appetizers. Broil 2 minutes; turn. Baste and broil 2 minutes; turn again. Baste and broil 1 minute or until bacon is browned.

CITRUS-MARINATED OLIVES
Makes 16 servings

1 cup (about 8 ounces) large green olives, drained

1 cup kalamata olives, rinsed and drained

⅓ cup extra virgin olive oil

¼ cup orange juice

3 tablespoons sherry vinegar or red wine vinegar

2 tablespoons lemon juice

1 tablespoon grated orange peel

1 tablespoon grated lemon peel

½ teaspoon ground cumin

¼ teaspoon red pepper flakes

Combine olives, oil, orange juice, vinegar, lemon juice, orange peel, lemon peel, cumin and red pepper flakes in medium glass bowl; toss to coat olives. Let stand overnight at room temperature. May be refrigerated up to 2 weeks.

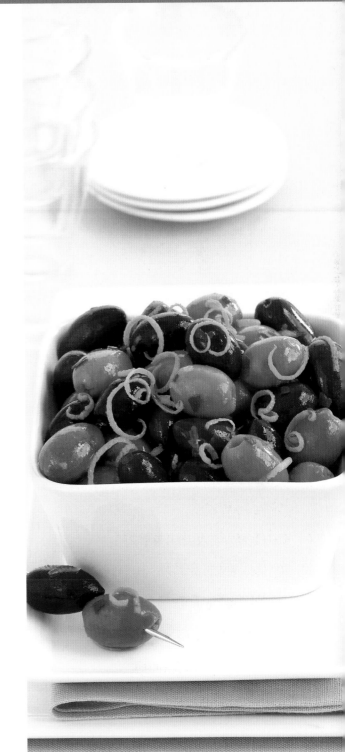

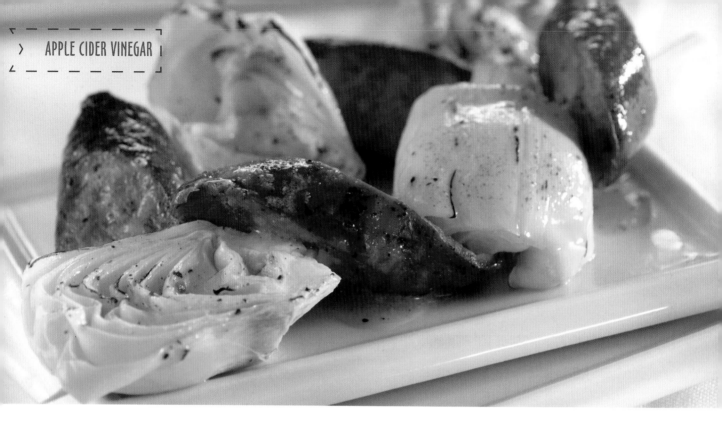

CHORIZO AND ARTICHOKE KABOBS WITH MUSTARD VINAIGRETTE

Makes 6 servings

1   can (about 14 ounces) large artichoke hearts, drained

2   (3-ounce) fully cooked chorizo-flavored chicken sausages or andouille sausages

3   tablespoons olive oil

2   teaspoons apple cider vinegar

1   teaspoon Dijon mustard

    Salt and black pepper

1. Preheat broiler. Line baking sheet or broiler pan with heavy-duty foil. Soak wooden skewers in warm water 20 minutes.

2. Cut artichoke hearts in half. Cut each sausage diagonally into 6 slices. Arrange 2 artichoke pieces and 2 sausage slices on each of 6 wooden skewers. Arrange skewers on prepared baking sheet. Broil 4 inches from heat 4 minutes or until artichokes are hot and sausage is browned.

3. Whisk oil, vinegar and mustard in small bowl. Season with salt and pepper. Serve with kabobs.

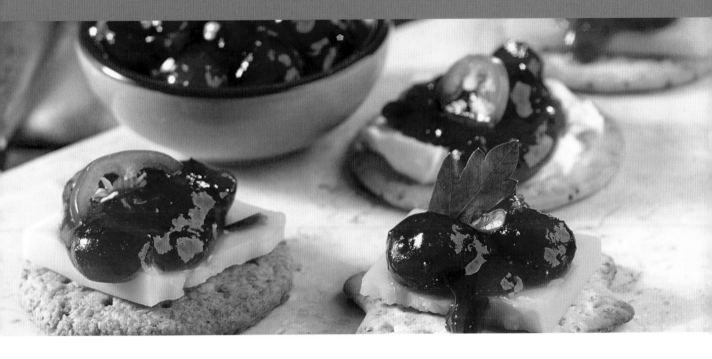

HOT PEPPER CRANBERRY JELLY APPETIZER

Makes 16 appetizer servings

½ cup whole berry cranberry sauce

¼ cup apricot fruit spread

1 teaspoon sugar

1 teaspoon apple cider vinegar

½ teaspoon red pepper flakes

½ teaspoon grated fresh ginger

Assorted crackers

Sliced cheeses

1. Combine cranberry sauce, fruit spread, sugar, vinegar and red pepper flakes in small saucepan. Cook and stir over medium heat until sugar is dissolved. **Do not boil.** Transfer to bowl; cool completely. Stir in ginger.

2. To serve, top crackers with cheese slices and spoonful of cranberry mixture.

SIPPABLE GAZPACHO
Makes 2 servings

- 2 small celery stalks
- 2 green onions, trimmed
- ½ cup cucumber slices
- 3 cups vegetable juice
- 1 tablespoon lemon juice
- 1 tablespoon red wine vinegar
- 1 teaspoon Worcestershire sauce
- 1 teaspoon hot pepper sauce
- ½ teaspoon ground cumin
- ⅛ teaspoon black pepper

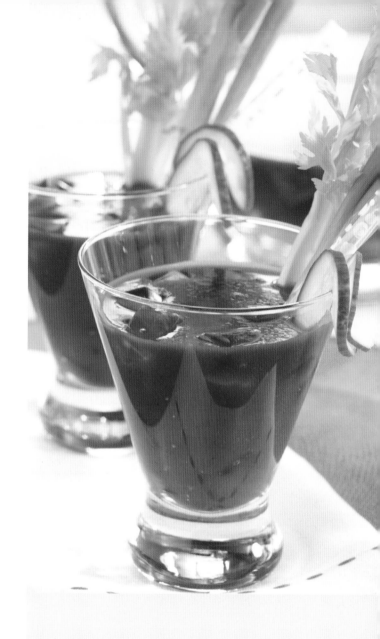

1. Place 1 celery stalk and 1 green onion in each of 2 glasses. Cut halfway into center of each cucumber slice; place on rim of each glass. Fill each glass with ice; set aside.

2. Stir together vegetable juice, lemon juice, vinegar, Worcestershire sauce, pepper sauce, cumin and pepper in pitcher. Pour into prepared glasses. Serve immediately.

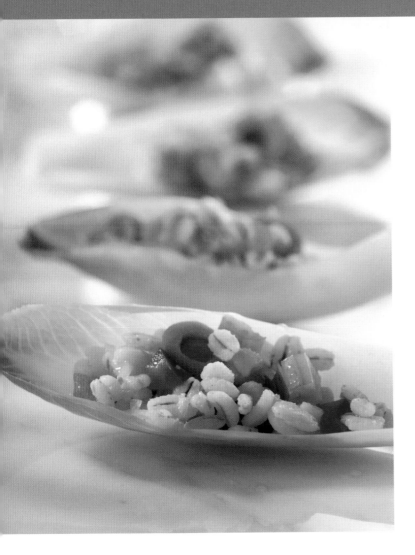

BARLEY "CAVIAR"
Makes 8 appetizers

4   cups water

½   teaspoon salt, divided

¾   cup uncooked pearl barley

½   cup sliced pimiento-stuffed olives

½   cup finely chopped red bell pepper

1   stalk celery, chopped

1   large shallot, finely chopped

1   jalapeño pepper,* minced *or* ¼ teaspoon red pepper flakes

2   tablespoons plus 1 teaspoon olive oil

4   teaspoons apple cider vinegar

¼   teaspoon ground cumin

⅛   teaspoon black pepper

8   leaves endive or Bibb lettuce

1. Bring water and ¼ teaspoon salt to a boil in medium saucepan over high heat. Stir in barley. Reduce heat to low. Cover and simmer 45 minutes or until barley is tender. Remove from heat; let stand 5 minutes. Rinse under cold water; drain well. Place in large bowl.

2. Stir in olives, bell pepper, celery, shallot and jalapeño pepper. Combine oil, vinegar, remaining ¼ teaspoon salt, cumin and black pepper in small bowl; stir to blend. Pour over barley mixture; stir gently to mix well. Let stand 10 minutes. To serve, spoon barley mixture evenly into endive leaves.

*Jalapeño peppers can sting and irritate the skin, so wear rubber gloves when handling peppers and do not touch your eyes.

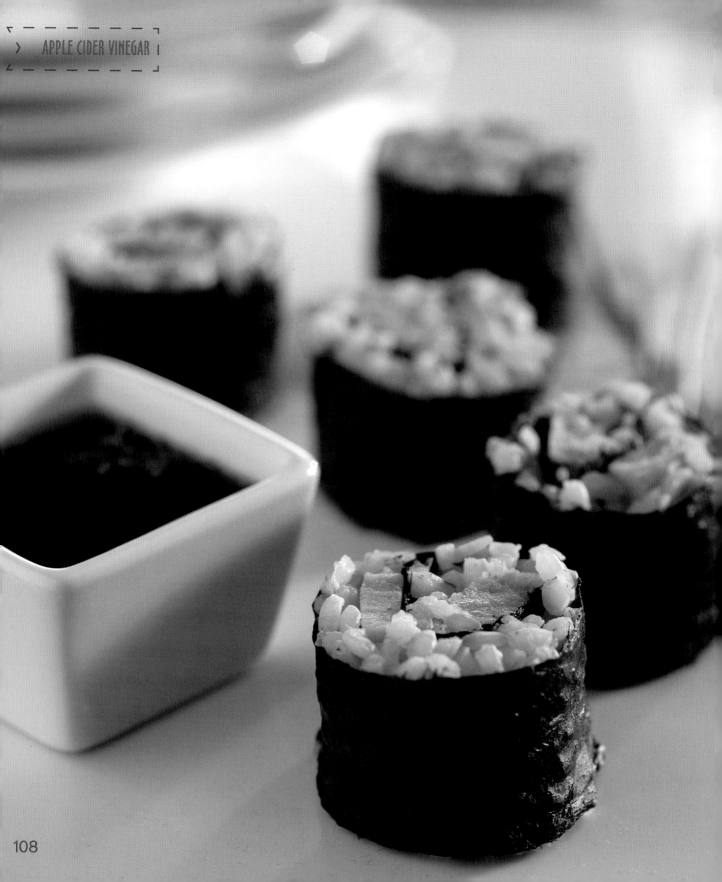

CALIFORNIA HAM ROLLS

Makes 4 servings

- 2 cups water
- ½ teaspoon salt, divided
- 1 cup short grain brown rice
- 2 tablespoons apple cider vinegar
- 1 tablespoon sugar
- 4 (8-inch) sheets sushi nori*
- 8 thin strips ham (about 4 ounces)
- ¼ cup soy sauce
- 1 tablespoon mirin (sweet rice wine)*
- 1 tablespoon minced chives (optional)

*May be found in the Asian section of your supermarket.

1. Bring water and ¼ teaspoon salt to a boil in medium saucepan over high heat. Stir in rice. Reduce heat to low. Cover and simmer 40 to 45 minutes or until water is absorbed and rice is tender but chewy. Spoon rice into large shallow bowl.

2. Combine vinegar, sugar and remaining ¼ teaspoon salt in small bowl. Microwave on HIGH 30 seconds. Stir to dissolve sugar. Pour over rice; stir to mix well. Set aside to cool.

3. Place 1 sheet of nori on work surface. Loosely spread about ½ cup rice over nori, leaving ½-inch border. Place 2 strips of ham along width of nori. Moisten top edge of nori sheet. Roll up tightly. Gently press to redistribute rice, if necessary. Cut into 6 slices with sharp knife. Place cut side up on serving plate. Repeat with remaining nori, rice and ham.

4. Combine soy sauce and mirin in small bowl; serve with ham rolls. Garnish with chives.

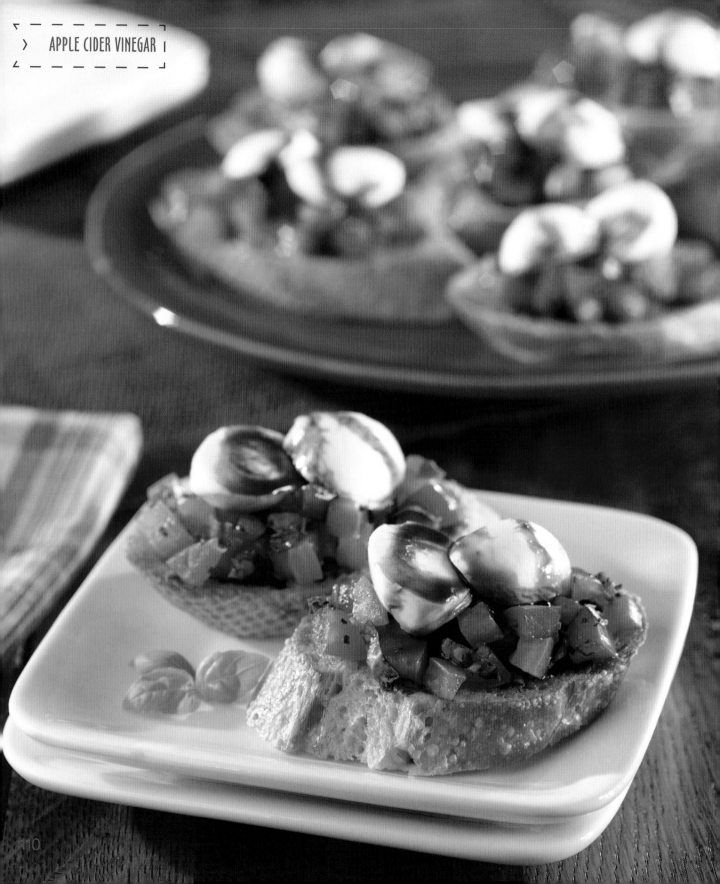

CAPRESE BRUSCHETTA
Makes 12 servings

¼ cup apple cider vinegar

2 tablespoons cola beverage

 Garlic powder

6 plum tomatoes, seeded and diced

12 large fresh basil leaves, chopped

¼ cup extra-virgin olive oil emulsified*
 with 1 tablespoon cola beverage

 Salt and black pepper

1 French baguette, cut into 24 slices

¼ cup (½ stick) butter, softened

12 small balls fresh mozzarella cheese, cut in half**

 Chopped fresh basil

*To emulsify means to blend two or more unblendable substances such as vinegar and oil. This can easily be done with a whisk, hand blender, or food processor.

**If unavailable, you may use an 8-ounce fresh mozzarella ball. Cut ball in quarters and slice each quarter into 6 slices, making 24 slices total.

1. Bring vinegar, cola and pinch of garlic powder to a boil over medium-high heat in small saucepan. Reduce heat to medium-low. Cook 10 to 15 minutes or until mixture is reduced to a syrup. Remove mixture from heat to cool.

2. Meanwhile, lightly toss tomatoes with chopped basil in medium bowl. Stir in emulsified oil, cola, salt and pepper.

3. Spread baguette slices with butter; sprinkle lightly with garlic powder. Toast baguette slices on baking sheet under broiler about 1 minute on each side or until crisp. To serve, top bread slices with 1 heaping tablespoon of tomato/basil mixture and 2 cheese halves. Drizzle with cooled syrup and garnish with basil.

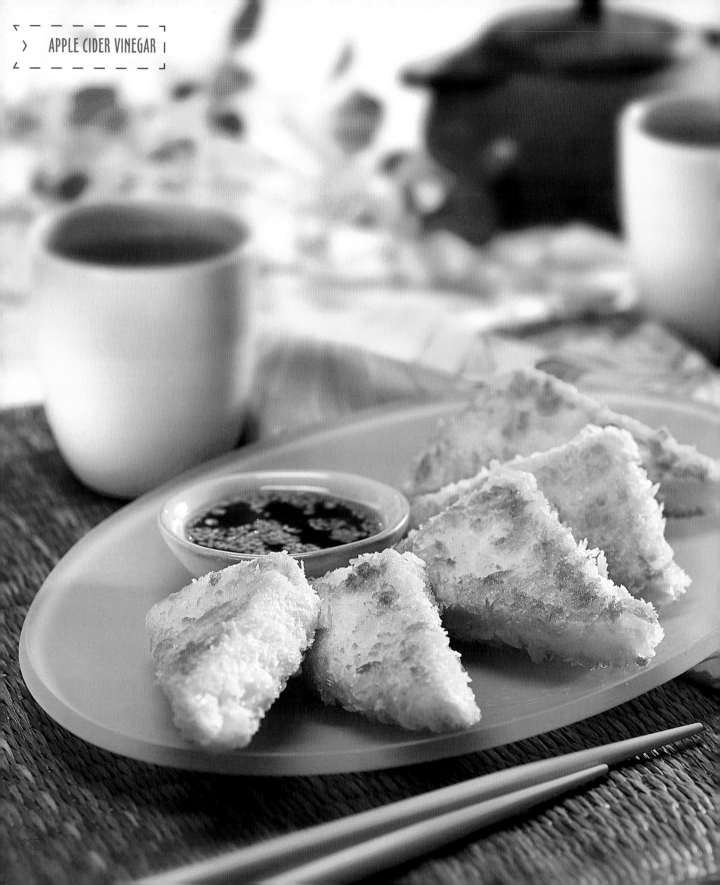

FRIED TOFU WITH SESAME DIPPING SAUCE
Makes 4 servings

- 3 tablespoons soy sauce or tamari
- 2 tablespoons unseasoned rice vinegar
- 2 teaspoons sugar
- 1 teaspoon sesame seeds, toasted*
- 1 teaspoon dark sesame oil
- 1/8 teaspoon red pepper flakes
- 1 package (about 14 ounces) extra firm tofu
- 2 tablespoons all-purpose flour
- 1 egg
- 1/4 cup panko bread crumbs**
- 4 tablespoons vegetable oil

*To toast sesame seeds, spread seeds in small skillet. Shake skillet over medium-low heat about 3 minutes or until seeds begin to pop and turn golden.

**Panko bread crumbs are used in Japanese cooking to provide a crisp exterior to fried foods. They are coarser than ordinary bread crumbs. Panko can be found in the Asian aisle of supermarkets.

1. Whisk soy sauce, vinegar, sugar, sesame seeds, sesame oil and red pepper flakes in small bowl until well blended; set aside.

2. Drain tofu and press between paper towels to remove excess water. Cut crosswise into four slices; cut each slice diagonally into triangles. Place flour in shallow dish. Beat egg in shallow bowl. Place panko in another shallow bowl.

3. Dip each piece of tofu in flour, turning to lightly coat all sides. Dip in egg, letting excess drip back into bowl. Roll in panko to coat.

4. Heat 2 tablespoons vegetable oil in large non-stick skillet over high heat. Reduce heat to medium; add half of tofu in single layer. Cook 1 to 2 minutes per side or until golden brown. Repeat with remaining tofu. Serve with sauce for dipping.

113

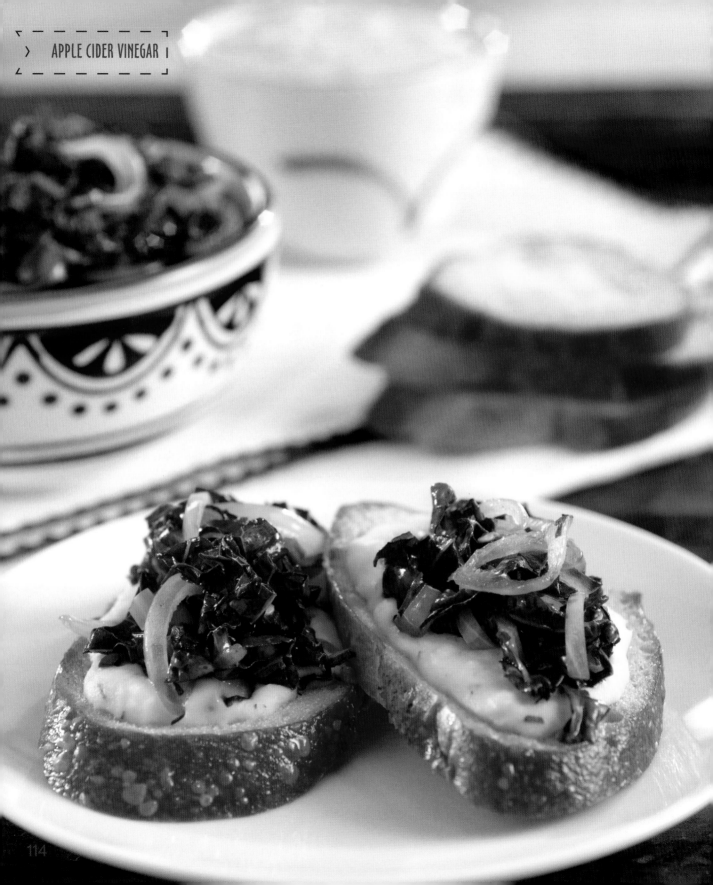

BEANS AND GREENS CROSTINI
Makes about 24 crostini

- 4 tablespoons olive oil, divided
- 1 small onion, thinly sliced
- 4 cups thinly sliced Italian black kale or other dinosaur kale variety
- 2 tablespoons minced garlic, divided
- 1 tablespoon apple cider vinegar
- 2 teaspoons salt, divided
- ¼ teaspoon red pepper flakes
- 1 can (about 15 ounces) cannellini beans, rinsed and drained
- 1 tablespoon chopped fresh rosemary
- Toasted baguette slices

1. Heat 1 tablespoon oil in large skillet over medium heat. Add onion; cook and stir 5 minutes or until softened. Add kale and 1 tablespoon garlic; cook 15 minutes or until kale is softened and most liquid has evaporated, stirring occasionally. Stir in vinegar, 1 teaspoon salt and red pepper flakes.

2. Meanwhile, combine beans, remaining 3 tablespoons oil, 1 tablespoon garlic, 1 teaspoon salt and rosemary in food processor or blender; process until smooth.

3. Spread baguette slices with bean mixture; top with kale.

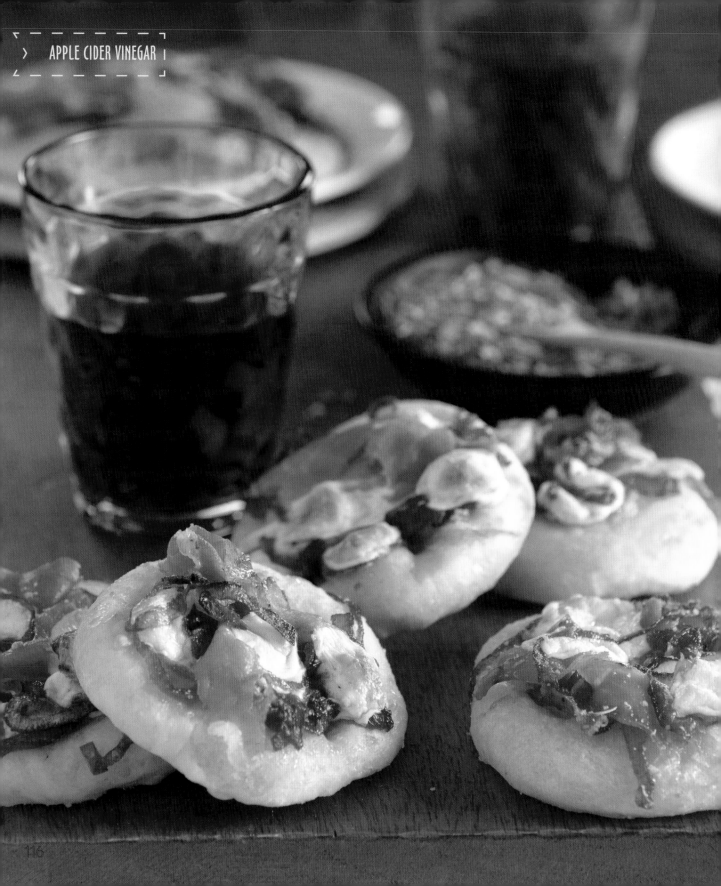

BALSAMIC ONION AND PROSCIUTTO PIZZETTES
Makes 16 pizzettes

- 1 package (16 ounces) refrigerated pizza dough*
- 2 tablespoons extra virgin olive oil, divided
- 1 large or 2 small red onions, cut in half and thinly sliced
- ¼ teaspoon salt
- 1½ tablespoons balsamic vinegar
- ⅛ teaspoon black pepper
- ⅓ cup grated Parmesan cheese
- 4 ounces fresh mozzarella, cut into small pieces
- 1 package (about 3 ounces) thinly sliced prosciutto, cut or torn into small pieces

*Frozen pizza dough can also be used. Thaw according to package directions.

1. Remove dough from refrigerator; let rest at room temperature while preparing onions. Heat 1 tablespoon oil in medium skillet over medium-high heat. Add onion and salt; cook 20 minutes or until tender and golden brown, stirring occasionally. Add vinegar and pepper; cook and stir 2 minutes. Set aside to cool.

2. Preheat oven to 450°F. Line two baking sheets with parchment paper.

3. Divide dough into 16 balls; press into 3-inch rounds (about ³/₈ inch thick) on prepared baking sheets. Brush each round with remaining 1 tablespoon oil; sprinkle with about 1 teaspoon Parmesan. Top with cooked onion, mozzarella, prosciutto and remaining Parmesan.

4. Bake 13 minutes or until crusts are golden brown.

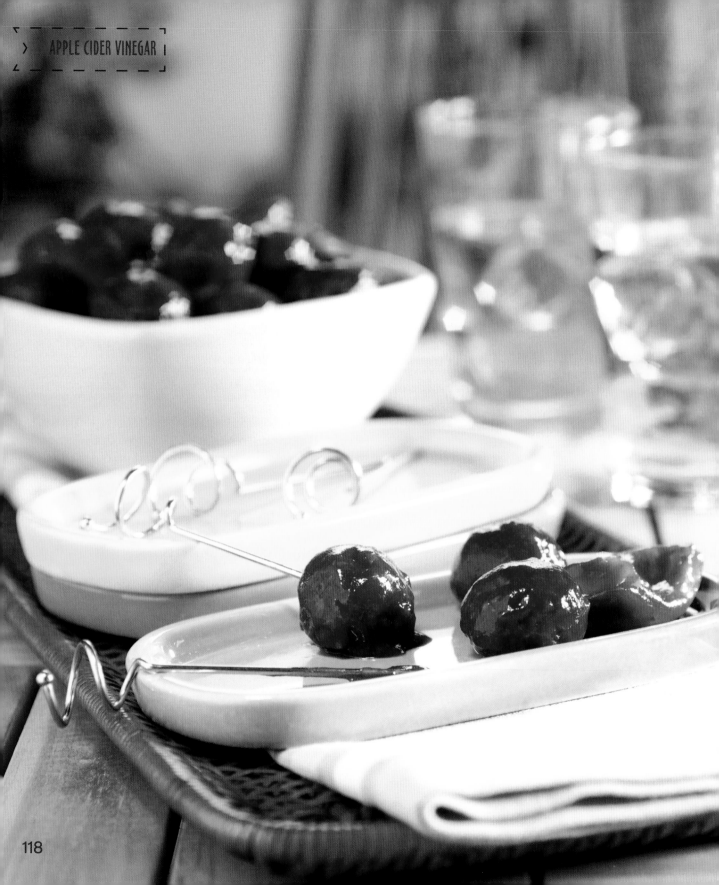

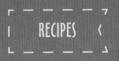

BARBECUED MEATBALLS
Makes about 4 dozen

- 2 pounds ground beef
- 1⅓ cups ketchup, divided
- 1 egg, lightly beaten
- 3 tablespoons seasoned dry bread crumbs
- 2 tablespoons dried onion flakes
- ¾ teaspoon garlic salt
- ½ teaspoon black pepper
- 1 cup packed brown sugar
- 1 can (6 ounces) tomato paste
- ¼ cup soy sauce
- ¼ cup apple cider vinegar
- 1½ teaspoons hot pepper sauce
  Chopped bell peppers (optional)

SLOW COOKER DIRECTIONS

1. Preheat oven to 350°F. Combine beef, ⅓ cup ketchup, egg, bread crumbs, onion flakes, garlic salt and black pepper in large bowl; mix well. Shape into 1-inch meatballs.

2. Arrange meatballs in single layer on two 15X10-inch jelly-roll pans. Bake 18 minutes or until browned. Transfer meatballs to slow cooker.

3. Combine remaining 1 cup ketchup, brown sugar, tomato paste, soy sauce, vinegar and hot pepper sauce in medium bowl; stir to blend. Pour over meatballs. Cover; cook on LOW 4 hours. Serve with cocktail picks. Garnish with bell peppers, if desired.

BARBECUED FRANKS: Arrange two (12-ounce) packages or three (8-ounce) packages cocktail franks in slow cooker. Prepare ketchup mixture as as directed in step 3; pour over franks. Cover; cook on LOW 4 hours.

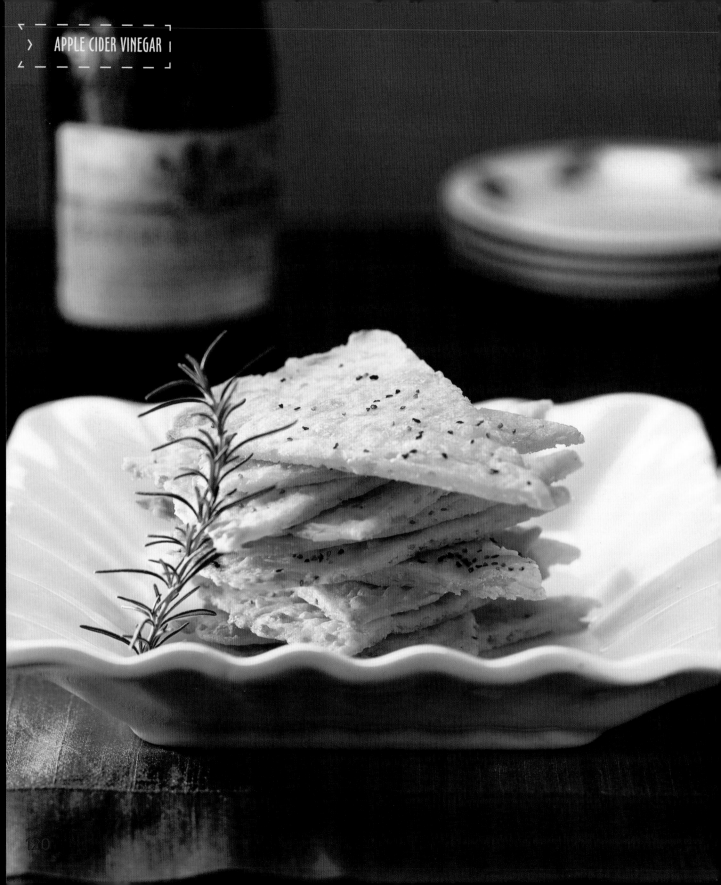

CHEDDAR CRISPS

Makes 32 crisps

~~~~~~

- 1¾ cups all-purpose flour
- ½ cup yellow cornmeal
- ¾ teaspoon sugar
- ¾ teaspoon salt
- ½ teaspoon baking soda
- ½ cup (1 stick) butter
- 1½ cups (6 ounces) shredded sharp Cheddar cheese
- ½ cup cold water
- 2 tablespoons apple cider vinegar
  Coarsely ground black pepper

1. Combine flour, cornmeal, sugar, salt and baking soda in large bowl. Cut in butter with pastry blender or two knives until mixture resembles coarse crumbs. Stir in cheese, water and vinegar with fork until mixture forms soft dough. Cover dough; refrigerate 1 hour or freeze 30 minutes until firm.*

2. Preheat oven to 375°F. Grease 2 baking sheets. Divide dough into 4 pieces. Roll each piece into paper-thin circle, about 13 inches in diameter, on floured surface. Sprinkle with pepper; press pepper firmly into dough.

3. Cut each circle into 8 wedges; place on prepared baking sheets. Bake 10 minutes or until crisp. Store in airtight container up to 3 days.

*To prepare frozen dough, thaw in the refrigerator before proceeding as directed.

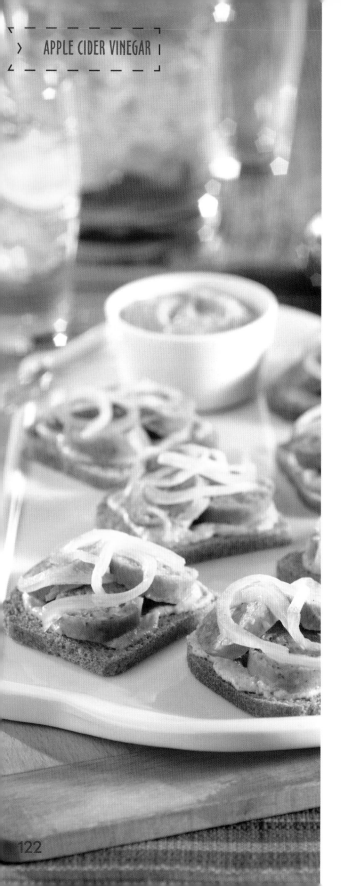

BRATS IN BEER

Makes 30 to 36 appetizers

1½ pounds bratwurst (about 5 or 6 links)

1   bottle (12 ounces) amber ale

1   onion, thinly sliced

2   tablespoons packed brown sugar

2   tablespoons apple cider vinegar

     Spicy brown mustard

     Cocktail rye bread

SLOW COOKER DIRECTIONS

1. Combine bratwurst, ale, onion, brown sugar and vinegar in slow cooker. Cover; cook on LOW 4 to 5 hours.

2. Remove bratwurst and onion slices from slow cooker. Cut bratwurst into ½-inch-thick slices. For mini open-faced sandwiches, spread mustard on cocktail rye bread. Top with bratwurst slices and onion.

TIP: Choose a light-tasting beer for cooking brats. Hearty ales might leave the meat tasting slightly bitter.

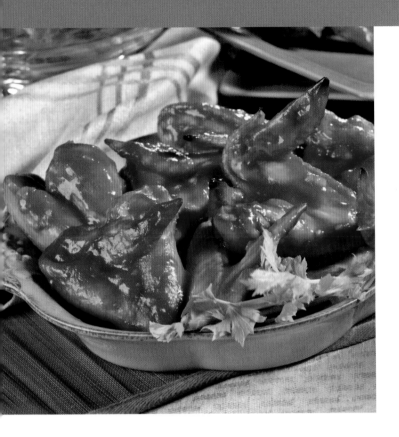

ANGEL WINGS
Makes 4 servings

1   can (10¾ ounces) condensed tomato soup, undiluted

¾   cup water

¼   cup packed brown sugar

2½ tablespoons apple cider vinegar

2   tablespoons chopped shallots

12 chicken wings

SLOW COOKER DIRECTIONS

1. Combine soup, water, brown sugar, vinegar and shallots in slow cooker; stir to blend.

2. Add chicken wings; turn to coat. Cover; cook on LOW 5 to 6 hours or until cooked through.

SOUPS, STEWS AND CHILIES

HOT AND SOUR SOUP
Makes 7 servings

3   cans (14½ ounces each) chicken broth

8   ounces boneless skinless chicken breasts, cut into ¼-inch-thick strips

1   cup shredded carrots

1   cup thinly sliced mushrooms

½   cup bamboo shoots, cut into matchstick-size strips

2   tablespoons rice vinegar or white wine vinegar

½ to ¾ teaspoon white pepper

¼ to ½ teaspoon hot pepper sauce

2   tablespoons cornstarch

2   tablespoons soy sauce

1   tablespoon dry sherry

2   medium green onions, sliced

1   egg, lightly beaten

1. Combine broth, chicken, carrots, mushrooms, bamboo shoots, vinegar, white pepper and hot pepper sauce in large saucepan; stir to blend. Bring to a boil over medium-high heat. Reduce heat to low. Cover and simmer 5 minutes or until chicken is no longer pink.

2. Combine cornstarch, soy sauce and sherry in small bowl; stir until smooth. Whisk cornstarh mixture into chicken broth mixture. Cook and stir until mixture comes to a boil. Stir in green onions and egg. Cook about 1 minute, stirring in one direction, until egg is cooked.

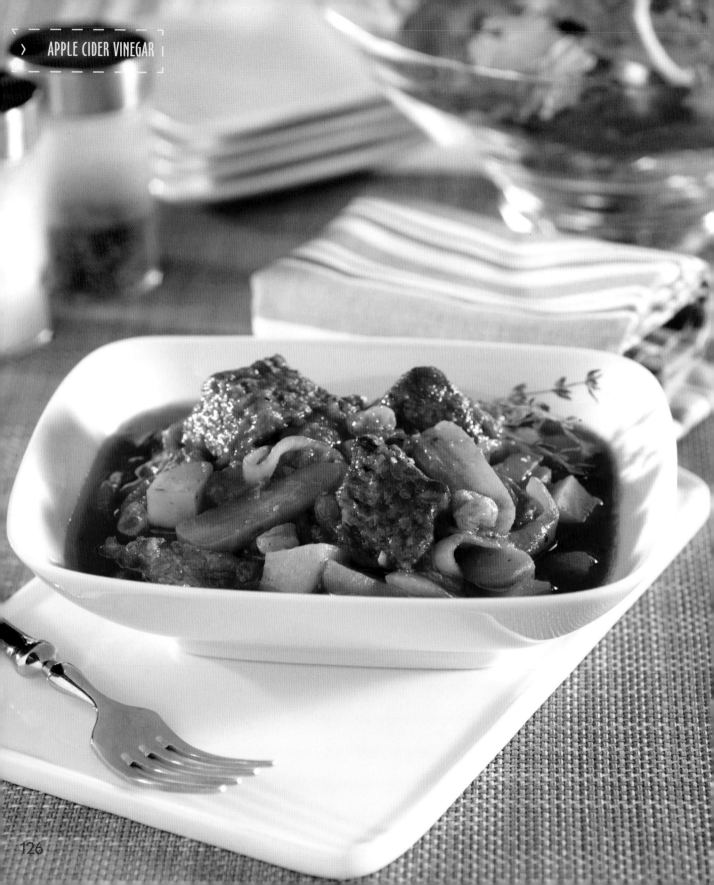

BEEF STEW WITH MOLASSES AND RAISINS

Makes 6 to 8 servings

- ⅓ cup all-purpose flour
- 2 teaspoons salt, divided
- 1½ teaspoons black pepper, divided
- 2 pounds boneless beef chuck roast, cut into 1½-inch pieces
- 5 tablespoons oil, divided
- 2 medium onions, sliced
- 1 can (28 ounces) diced tomatoes, drained
- 1 cup beef broth
- 3 tablespoons molasses
- 2 tablespoons apple cider vinegar
- 4 cloves garlic, minced
- 2 teaspoons dried thyme
- 1 teaspoon celery salt
- 1 bay leaf
- 1 small package (8 ounces) baby carrots, cut into halves lengthwise
- 2 parsnips, diced
- ½ cup golden raisins

SLOW COOKER DIRECTIONS

1. Combine flour, 1½ teaspoons salt and 1 teaspoon pepper in large bowl; stir to blend. Toss beef in flour mixture. Heat 2 tablespoons oil in large skillet or Dutch oven over medium-high heat. Add half of beef; cook 6 to 8 minutes or until browned on all sides. Remove browned beef to large plate. Repeat with 2 tablespoons oil and remaining beef.

2. Add remaining 1 tablespoon oil to skillet. Add onions; cook and stir 5 minutes, scraping up any browned bits from bottom of skillet. Add tomatoes, broth, molasses, vinegar, garlic, thyme, celery salt, bay leaf and remaining ½ teaspoon salt and ½ teaspoon pepper. Bring to a boil. Add browned beef; boil 1 minute.

3. Remove mixture to slow cooker. Cover; cook on LOW 5 hours or on HIGH 2½ hours. Stir in carrots, parsnips and raisins. Cover; cook 1 to 2 hours on HIGH or until vegetables are tender. Remove and discard bay leaf.

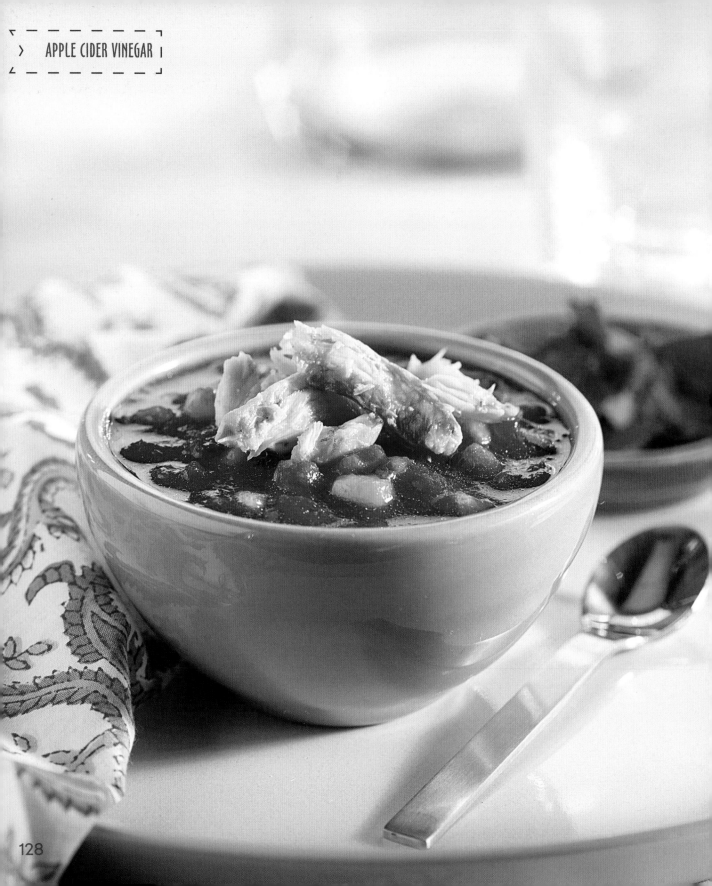

CORN AND CRAB GAZPACHO
Makes 6 servings

- 1 cucumber, peeled, seeded and coarsely chopped
- 3 green onions, coarsely chopped
- 2 tablespoons coarsely chopped fresh Italian parsley or cilantro
- 2 pounds grape or cherry tomatoes
- 3 cups tomato juice, chilled
- 1 cup cooked fresh corn (1 large ear) *or* 1 cup thawed frozen corn
- 3 tablespoons olive oil
- 2 tablespoons red wine vinegar
- 1¼ teaspoons red pepper flakes
- 1 teaspoon salt
- ¼ teaspoon black pepper
- 1½ cups flaked cooked crabmeat (about 8 ounces) *or* 8 ounces cooked baby shrimp

1. Combine cucumber, green onions and parsley in food processor. Process using on/off pulsing action until finely chopped. Remove to large pitcher or bowl. Add tomatoes to food processor. Process using on/off pulsing action until finely chopped. Add to cucumber mixture.

2. Stir tomato juice, corn, oil, vinegar, red pepper flakes, salt and black pepper. Cover; refrigerate 1 to 3 hours.

3. Pour gazpacho into 6 bowls. Top each serving with ¼ cup crabmeat.

NOTE: Gazpacho can be made several hours in advance and chilled. Bring to room temperature before serving.

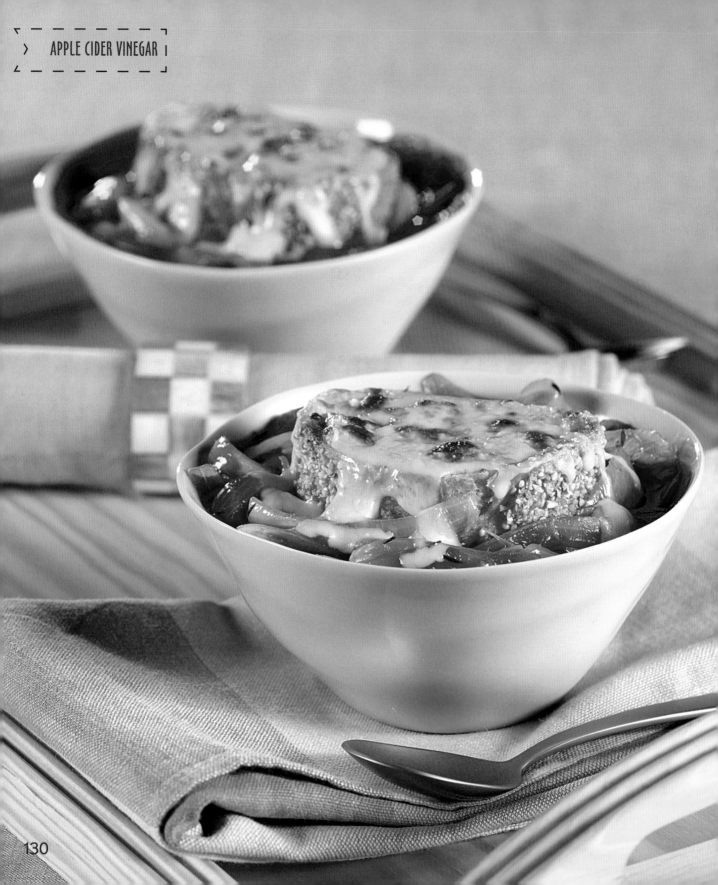

FRENCH ONION SOUP FOR DEUX

Makes 2 servings

- 2 teaspoons olive oil
- ¾ pound yellow onions, halved lengthwise and cut into thin strips
- 1 clove garlic, thinly sliced
  Salt and black pepper
- 1 cup chicken broth
- 1 cup water
- 1 tablespoon balsamic vinegar
- 1 whole bay leaf
- ½ teaspoon dried thyme
- 2 thick slices crusty, peasant-style, whole wheat bread
- ¼ cup (1 ounce) shredded white cheese, such as Muenster or Monterey-Jack

1. Heat oil in large saucepan over medium heat. Add onions and garlic; cook and stir 20 minutes or until onions are soft and golden brown. If onions start to stick or burn, reduce heat slightly and add water one tablespoon at a time. Sprinkle onions with salt and pepper.

2. Reduce heat to low. Add broth, water, vinegar, bay leaf and thyme; simmer until heated through. Remove and discard bay leaf.

3. Preheat broiler. Toast bread under broiler on both sides. To serve, ladle soup into two ovenproof bowls; top each with toasted bread. Sprinkle bread with cheese. Place bowls on baking sheet. Broil until cheese is melted and is bubbly and browned.

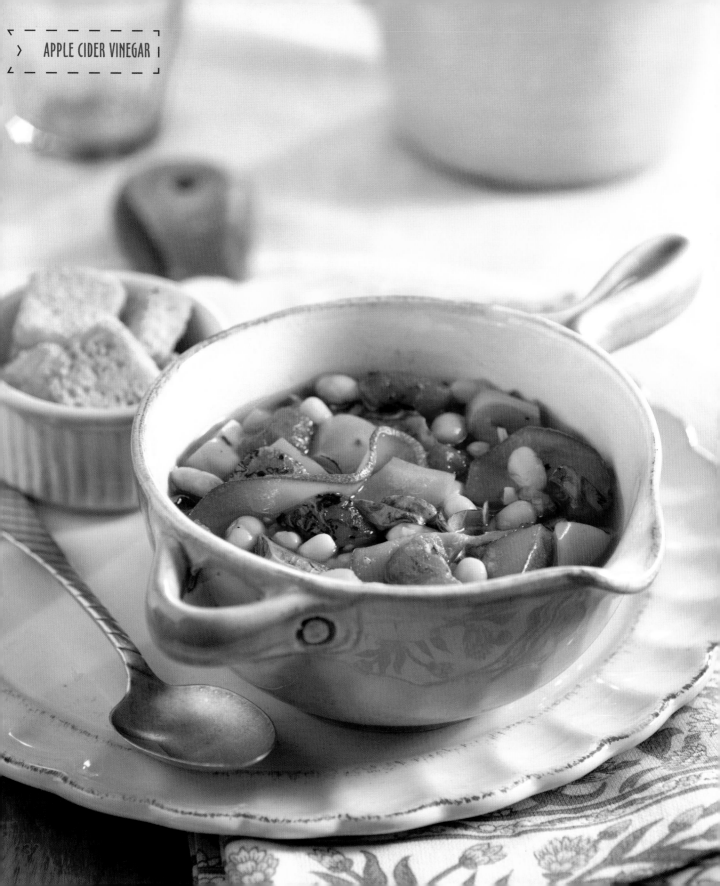

ITALIAN SKILLET ROASTED VEGETABLE SOUP
Makes 5 servings

- 2 tablespoons olive oil, divided
- 1 medium orange, red or yellow bell pepper, chopped
- 1 clove garlic, minced
- 2 cups water
- 1 can (about 14 ounces) diced tomatoes
- 1 medium zucchini, thinly sliced lengthwise
- 1/8 teaspoon red pepper flakes
- 1 can (about 15 ounces) navy beans, rinsed and drained
- 3 to 4 tablespoons chopped fresh basil
- 1 tablespoon balsamic vinegar
- 3/4 teaspoon salt
- 1/2 teaspoon liquid smoke (optional)
  Croutons (optional)

1. Heat 1 tablespoon oil in Dutch oven over medium-high heat. Add bell pepper; cook and stir 4 minutes or until edges are browned. Add garlic; cook and stir 15 seconds. Add water, tomatoes, zucchini and red pepper flakes; bring to a boil over high heat. Reduce heat to low. Cover and simmer 20 minutes.

2. Add beans, basil, remaining 1 tablespoon oil, vinegar, salt and liquid smoke, if desired; simmer 5 minutes. Remove from heat. Let stand, covered, 10 minutes before serving. Top with croutons, if desired.

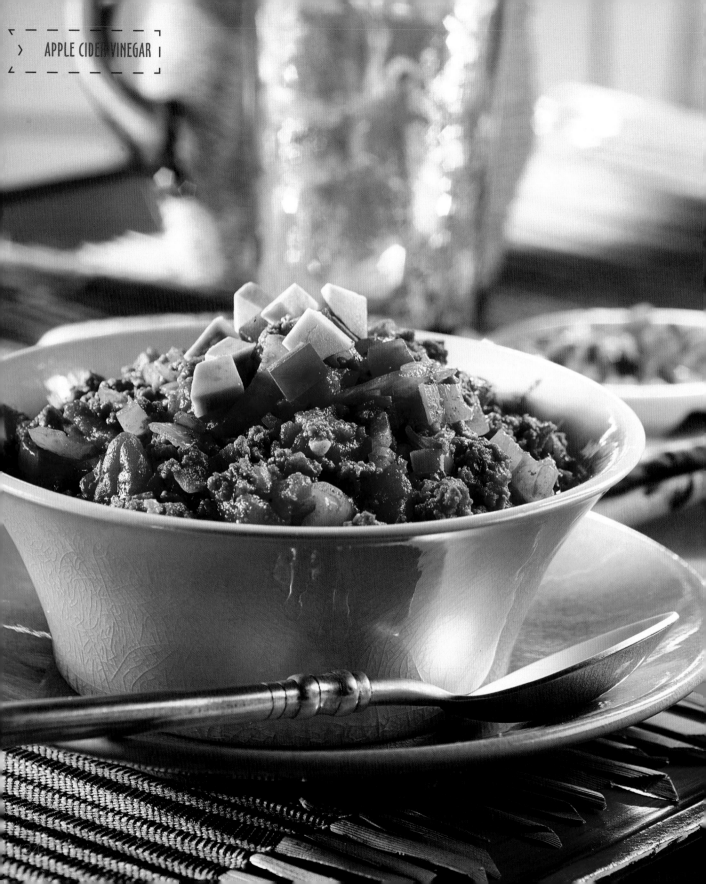

RED AND GREEN NO-BEAN CHILI

Makes 10 to 12 servings

4   pounds ground beef

2   large onions, chopped

3   banana peppers, seeded and sliced

¼   cup chili powder

2   tablespoons minced garlic

1   can (about 28 ounces) diced tomatoes with mild green chiles, undrained

1   can (about 14 ounces) beef broth

2   cans (4 ounces each) diced mild green chiles, drained

2   tablespoons ground cumin

2   tablespoons apple cider vinegar

1   to 2 tablespoons hot paprika

1   tablespoon dried oregano

Hot pepper sauce

Diced avocado and chopped red bell peppers (optional)

1. Brown beef in large skillet or Dutch oven over medium-high heat 6 to 8 minutes, stirring to break up meat. Drain fat. Stir in onions, banana peppers, chili powder and garlic. Reduce heat to medium-low; cook 30 minutes, stirring occasionally.

2. Add tomatoes with juice, broth, green chiles, cumin, vinegar, paprika, oregano and hot pepper sauce; cook and stir 30 minutes. Garnish with avocado and red bell peppers.

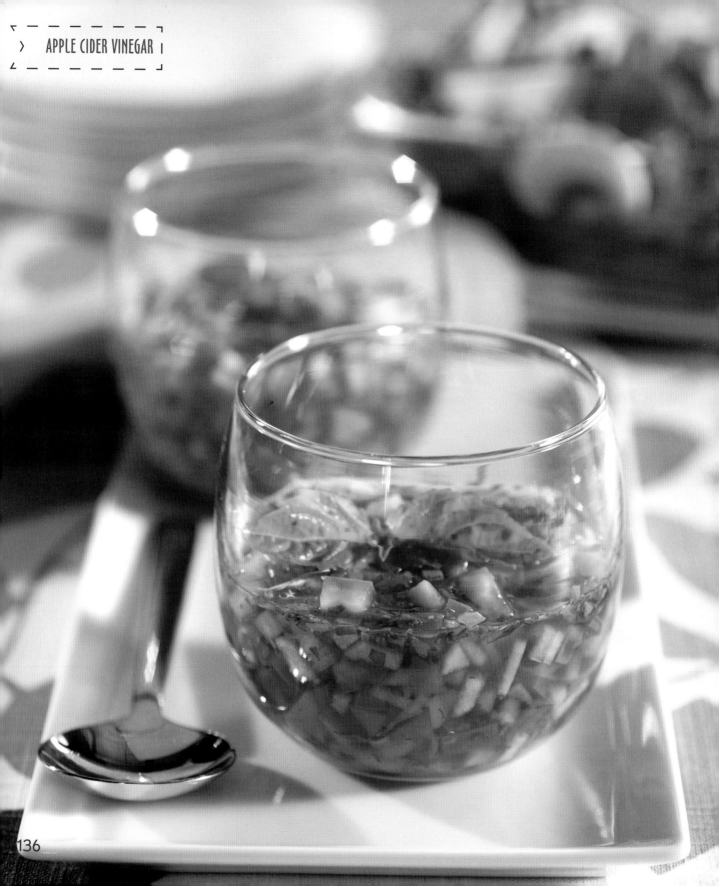

CHILLED FRESH TOMATO BASIL SOUP
Makes 4 servings

3   medium tomatoes, diced

1   cup finely chopped green bell pepper

1   cup water

½   medium cucumber, peeled, seeded and finely chopped

¼   cup chopped fresh basil

¼   cup finely chopped pepperoncini peppers

3   tablespoons red wine vinegar

2   tablespoons chopped fresh parsley

2   tablespoons extra virgin olive oil

½   teaspoon salt

Combine tomatoes, bell pepper, water, cucumber, basil, pepperoncini peppers, vinegar, parsley, oil and salt in medium bowl; stir to blend. Refrigerate 30 minutes or until chilled.

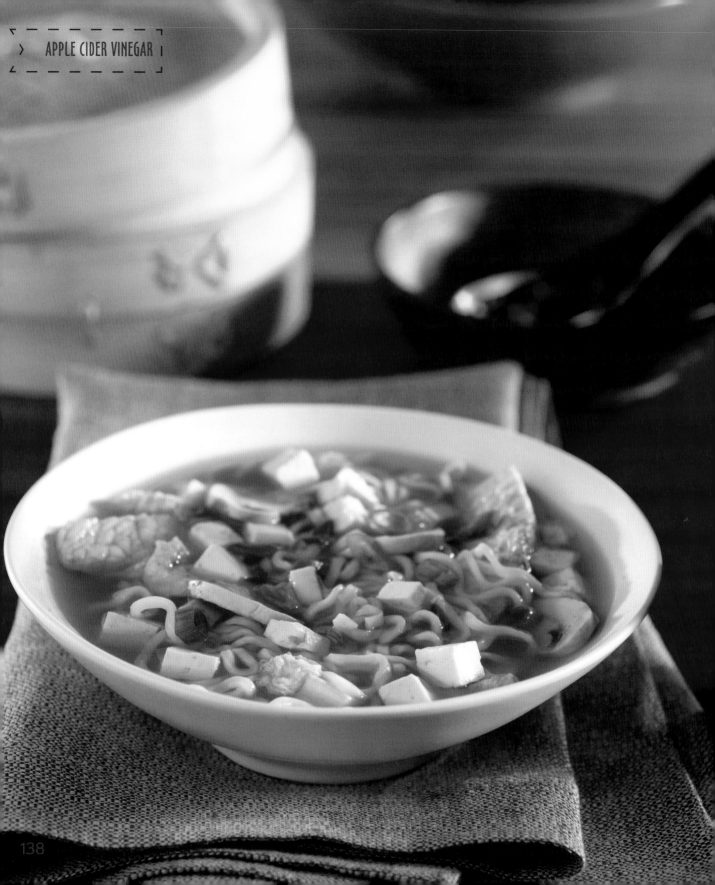

ASIAN RAMEN NOODLE SOUP

Makes 4 servings

2　cans (about 14 ounces each) chicken broth

4　ounces boneless pork loin, cut into thin strips

¾　cup thinly sliced mushrooms

½　cup firm tofu, cut into ¼-inch cubes (optional)

3　tablespoons white vinegar

3　tablespoons dry sherry

1　tablespoon soy sauce

½　teaspoon ground red pepper

1　package (3 ounces) ramen noodles, any flavor, broken*

1　egg, beaten

¼　cup finely chopped green onions, green tops only

*Discard seasoning packet or reserve for another use.

1. Bring broth to a boil in large saucepan over high heat; add pork, mushrooms and tofu, if desired. Reduce heat to medium-low. Simmer, covered, 5 minutes. Stir in vinegar, sherry, soy sauce and ground red pepper.

2. Return broth mixture to a boil over high heat. Stir in noodles; cook and stir 5 to 7 minutes or until noodles are tender. Slowly stir in egg and green onions; remove from heat. Ladle soup into individual bowls.

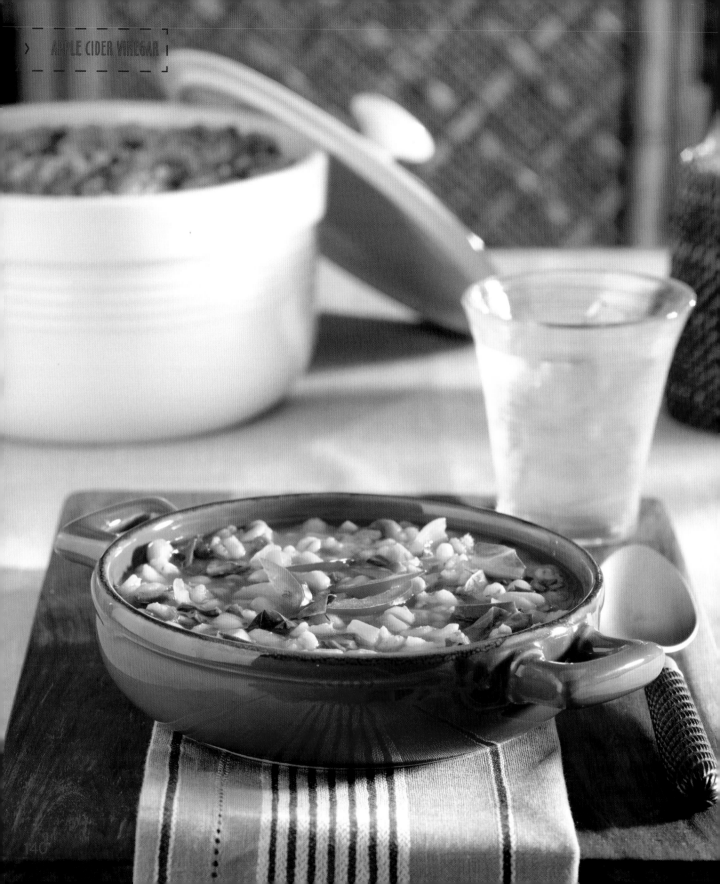

GREENS, WHITE BEAN AND BARLEY SOUP
Makes 8 servings

- 2 tablespoons olive oil
- 3 carrots, diced
- 1½ cups chopped onions
- 2 cloves garlic, minced
- 1½ cups sliced mushrooms
- 6 cups vegetable broth
- 2 cups cooked barley
- 1 can (about 15 ounces) Great Northern beans, rinsed and drained
- 2 bay leaves
- 1 teaspoon sugar
- 1 teaspoon dried thyme
- 7 cups chopped stemmed collard greens (about 24 ounces)
- 1 tablespoon white wine vinegar
  Hot pepper sauce
  Red bell pepper strips (optional)

1. Heat oil in Dutch oven over medium heat. Add carrots, onions and garlic; cook and stir 3 minutes. Add mushrooms; cook and stir 5 minutes or until carrots are tender.

2. Add broth, barley, beans, bay leaves, sugar and thyme. Bring to a boil over high heat. Reduce heat to medium-low. Cover and simmer 5 minutes. Add greens; simmer 10 minutes. Remove and discard bay leaves. Stir in vinegar. Season with hot pepper sauce. Garnish with red bell peppers.

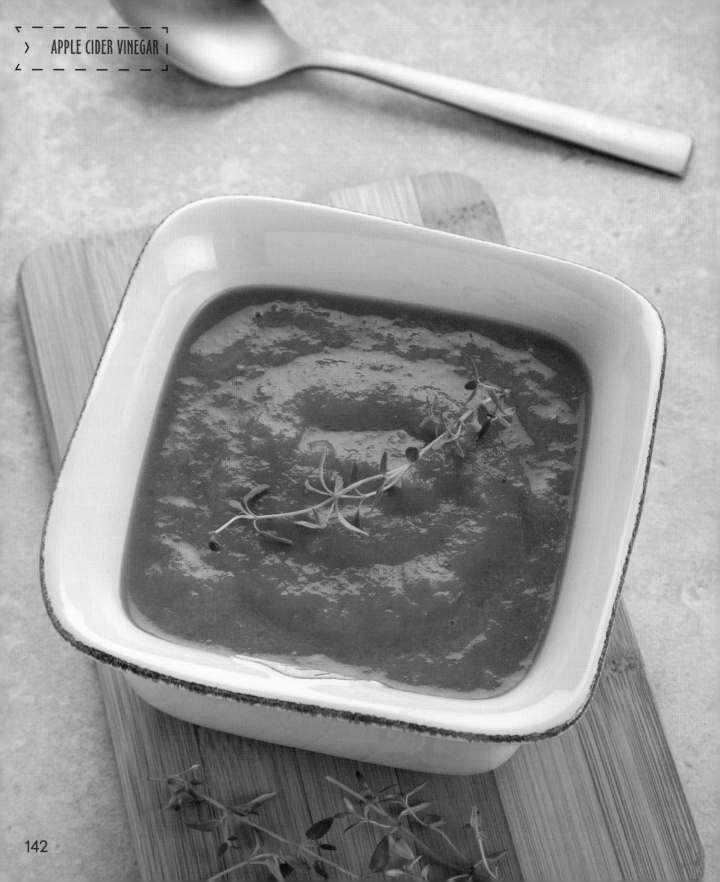

SWEET RED BELL PEPPER SOUP
Makes 8 servings

~~~~~~~~~~~~~~~~~~~~~~~~~~~~~~~~~~

8 red bell peppers, sliced into quarters

2 tablespoons olive oil

1 onion, thinly sliced

3 cloves garlic, minced

1 teaspoon black pepper

1 teaspoon dried oregano

2 tablespoons balsamic vinegar

2 teaspoons sugar

1½ tablespoons fresh thyme, divided

SLOW COOKER DIRECTIONS

1. Cut peppers in half and remove stem and seeds; slice into quarters. Coat inside of slow cooker with oil. Add bell peppers, onion, garlic, black pepper and oregano; gently mix. Cover; cook on HIGH 4 hours or until bell peppers are very tender; stirring halfway through cooking.

2. Purée soup in slow cooker using hand-held immersion blender or remove mixture in batches to blender or food processor. Blend until smooth. Stir in vinegar and sugar. Ladle soup into bowls; garnish with thyme.

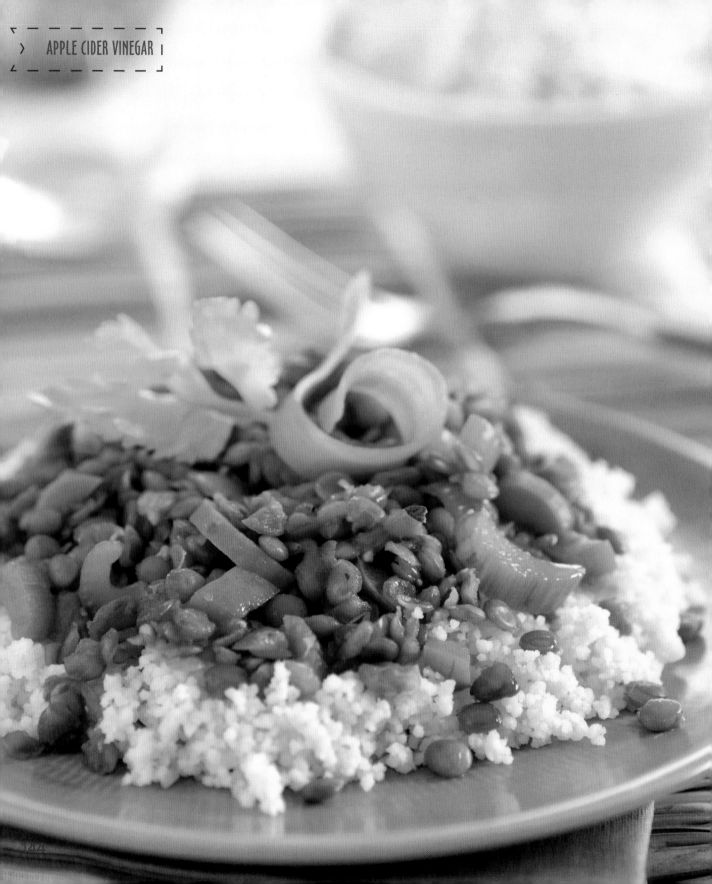

LENTIL STEW OVER COUSCOUS
Makes 12 servings

- 3 cups dried lentils (1 pound), sorted and rinsed
- 3 cups water
- 1 can (about 14 ounces) vegetable broth
- 1 can (about 14 ounces) diced tomatoes
- 1 large onion, chopped
- 1 green bell pepper, chopped
- 4 stalks celery, chopped
- 1 medium carrot, halved lengthwise and sliced
- 2 cloves garlic, chopped
- 1 teaspoon dried marjoram
- ¼ teaspoon black pepper
- 1 tablespoon olive oil
- 1 tablespoon apple cider vinegar
- 4½ to 5 cups hot cooked couscous or quinoa

SLOW COOKER DIRECTIONS

1. Combine lentils, water, broth, tomatoes, onion, bell pepper, celery, carrot, garlic, marjoram and black pepper in slow cooker; stir to blend. Cover; cook on LOW 8 to 9 hours.

2. Stir in oil and vinegar. Serve over couscous.

TIP: Lentil stew keeps well in the refrigerator up to 1 week. Stew can also be frozen in an airtight container up to three months.

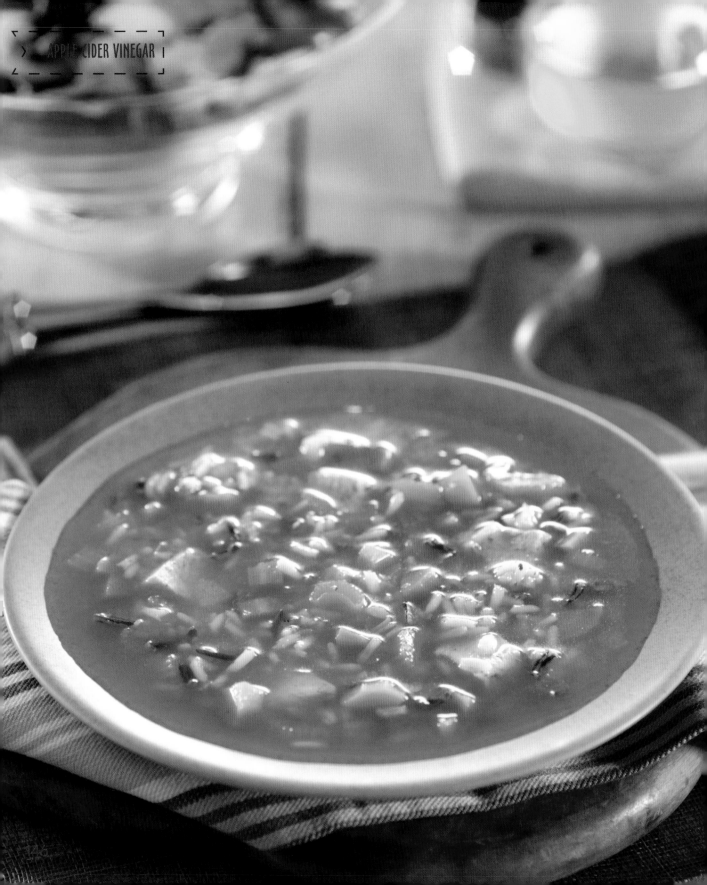

CHICKEN AND WILD RICE SOUP

Makes 9 servings

- 3 cans (about 14 ounces each) chicken broth
- 1 pound boneless skinless chicken breasts or thighs, cut into 1-inch pieces
- 2 cups water
- 1 cup sliced celery
- 1 cup diced carrots
- 1 package (6 ounces) converted long grain and wild rice mix with seasoning packet (not quick-cooking or instant rice)
- ½ cup chopped onion
- ½ teaspoon black pepper
- 2 teaspoons apple cider vinegar
- 1 tablespoon dried parsley flakes

SLOW COOKER DIRECTIONS

1. Combine broth, chicken, water, celery, carrots, rice with seasoning packet, onion and pepper in slow cooker; mix well.

2. Cover; cook on LOW 6 to 7 hours or on HIGH 4 to 5 hours or until chicken is tender.

3. Stir in vinegar. Sprinkle with parsley.

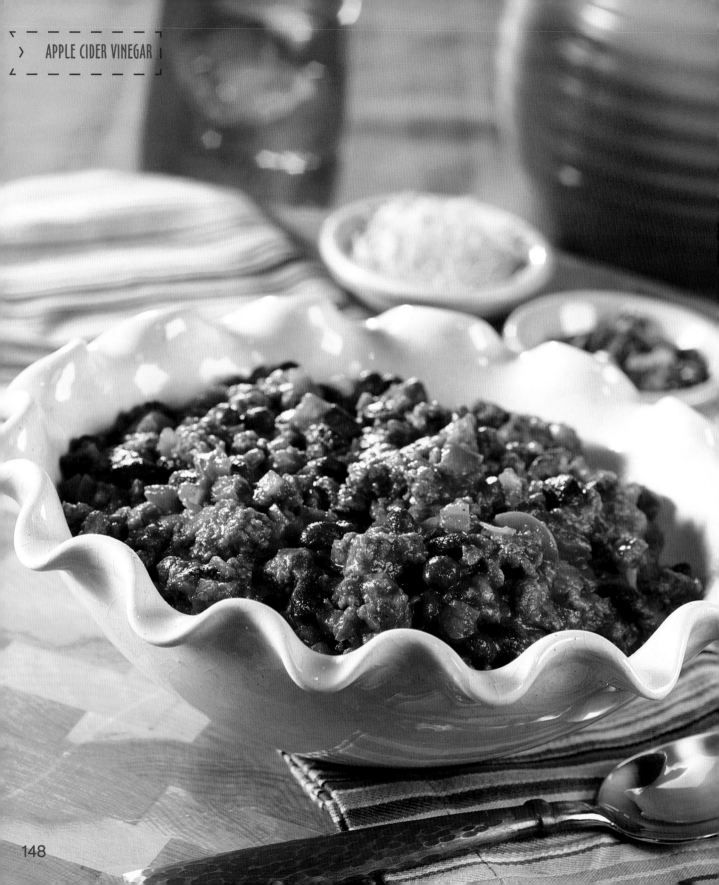

HEARTY CHILI WITH BLACK BEANS

Makes 4 servings

- 1   tablespoon vegetable oil
- 1   pound ground beef chuck
- 1   can (about 14 ounces) beef broth
- 1   large onion, minced
- 1   green bell pepper, seeded and diced
- 2   teaspoons chili powder
- ½   teaspoon ground allspice
- ¼   teaspoon cinnamon
- ¼   teaspoon paprika
- 1   can (about 15 ounces) black beans, rinsed and drained
- 1   can (about 14 ounces) crushed tomatoes
- 2   teaspoons apple cider vinegar

1. Heat oil in large skillet over medium-high heat. Add beef, broth, onion and bell pepper; cook 6 to 8 minutes, stirring to break up meat.

2. Stir in chili powder, allspice, cinnamon and paprika. Reduce heat to medium-low. Simmer 10 minutes. Stir in black beans, tomatoes and vinegar; bring to a boil.

3. Reduce heat to low. Simmer 20 to 25 minutes or until chili is thickened.

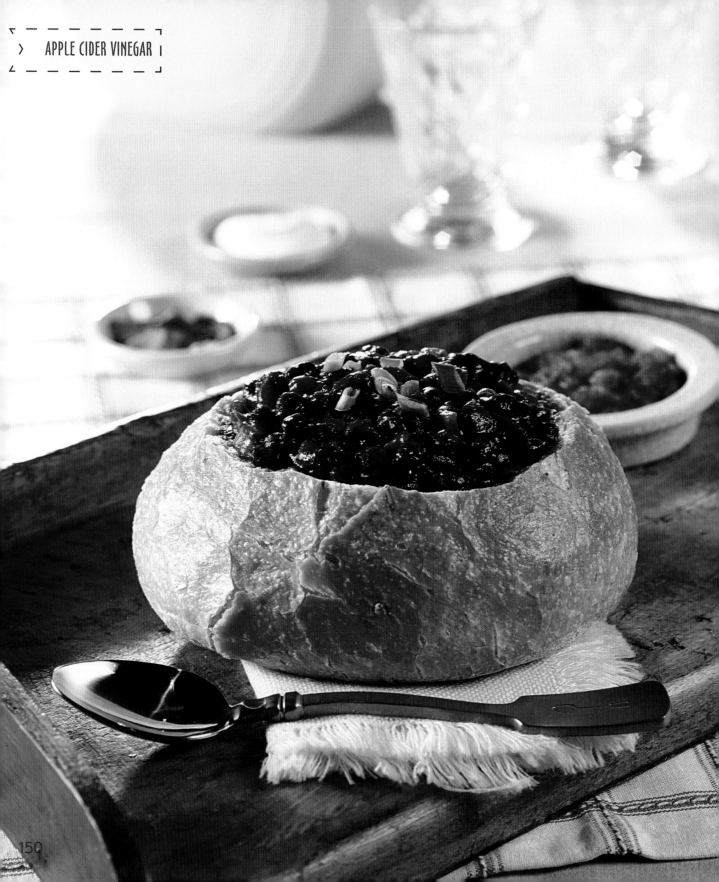

BLACK BEAN CHILI

Makes 6 servings

1   pound uncooked dried black beans

    Cold water

6   cups water

1   whole bay leaf

3   tablespoons vegetable oil

2   large onions, chopped

3   cloves garlic, minced

1   can (about 14 ounces) diced tomatoes

2   to 3 fresh or canned jalapeño peppers,
    * stemmed, seeded and minced

2   tablespoons chili powder

1½ teaspoons salt

1   teaspoon paprika

1   teaspoon dried oregano

1   teaspoon unsweetened cocoa powder

½   teaspoon ground cumin

¼   teaspoon ground cinnamon

1   tablespoon red wine vinegar

OPTIONAL TOPPINGS: plain yogurt or
sour cream, picante sauce and/or sliced green onions
or chopped fresh cilantro (optional)

*Jalapeño peppers can sting and irritate the skin,
so wear rubber gloves when handling peppers and
do not touch your eyes.

1. Sort beans, discarding any foreign material. Place beans in 8-quart Dutch oven. Add enough cold water to cover beans by 2 inches. Cover; bring to a boil over high heat. Boil 2 minutes. Remove from heat. Let soak, covered, 1 hour. Drain. Add 6 cups water and bay leaf to beans in Dutch oven. Return to heat. Bring to a boil. Reduce heat and simmer, partially covered, 1 to 2 hours or until tender.

2. Meanwhile, heat oil in large skillet over medium heat. Add onions and garlic; cook 3 to 4 minutes or until onions are tender. Add tomatoes, jalapeño peppers, chili powder, salt, paprika, oregano, cocoa, cumin and cinnamon. Simmer 15 minutes. Add tomato mixture to beans. Stir in vinegar. Continue simmering 30 minutes or until beans are very tender and chili has thickened slightly. Remove and discard bay leaf. Ladle chili into individual bowls. Serve with desired toppings.

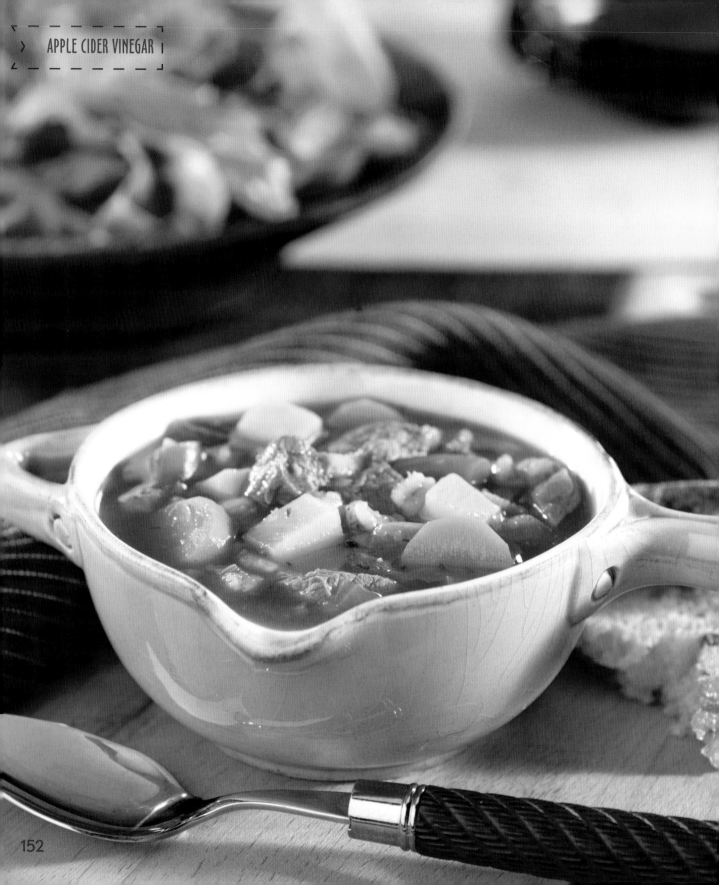

BEEF BARLEY SOUP

Makes 4 servings

Nonstick cooking spray

¾ pound boneless beef top round steak, trimmed and cut into ½-inch pieces

3 cans (about 14 ounces each) beef broth

2 cups unpeeled cubed potatoes

1 can (about 14 ounces) diced tomatoes

1 cup chopped onion

1 cup sliced carrots

½ cup uncooked pearl barley

1 tablespoon apple cider vinegar

2 teaspoons caraway seeds

2 teaspoons dried marjoram

2 teaspoons dried thyme

½ teaspoon salt

½ teaspoon black pepper

1½ cups sliced green beans (½-inch slices)

1. Spray large saucepan with cooking spray; heat over medium heat. Add beef; cook and stir 6 to 8 minutes or until browned on all sides.

2. Stir in broth, potatoes, tomatoes, onion, carrots, barley, vinegar, caraway seeds, marjoram, thyme, salt and pepper; bring to a boil over high heat. Reduce heat to low. Cover and simmer 1½ hours. Add green beans; cook, uncovered, 30 minutes or until beef is fork-tender.

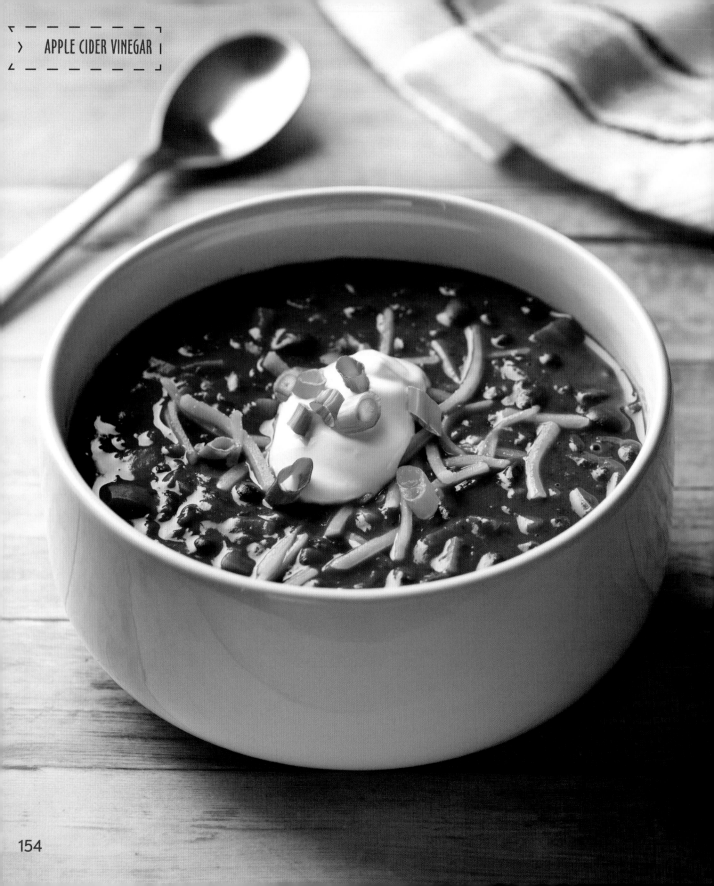

BLACK BEAN SOUP

Makes 4 to 6 servings

- 2   tablespoons vegetable oil
- 1   cup diced onion
- 1   stalk celery, diced
- 2   carrots, diced
- ½   small green bell pepper, diced
- 4   cloves garlic, minced
- 4   cans (15 ounces each) black beans, rinsed and drained, divided
- 4   cups (32 ounces) chicken or vegetable broth, divided
- 2   tablespoons apple cider vinegar
- 2   teaspoons chili powder
- ½   teaspoon salt
- ½   teaspoon ground red pepper
- ½   teaspoon ground cumin
- ¼   teaspoon liquid smoke

1. Heat oil in large saucepan or Dutch oven over medium-low heat. Add onion, celery, carrots, bell pepper and garlic; cook 10 minutes, stirring occasionally.

2. Combine half of beans and 1 cup broth in food processor or blender; process until smooth. Add to vegetables in saucepan.

3. Stir in remaining beans, broth, vinegar, chili powder, salt, ground red pepper, cumin and liquid smoke; bring to a boil over high heat. Reduce heat to medium-low. Cook 1 hour or until vegetables are tender and soup is thickened. Garnish as desired.

Optional toppings: sour cream, chopped green onions and shredded Cheddar cheese

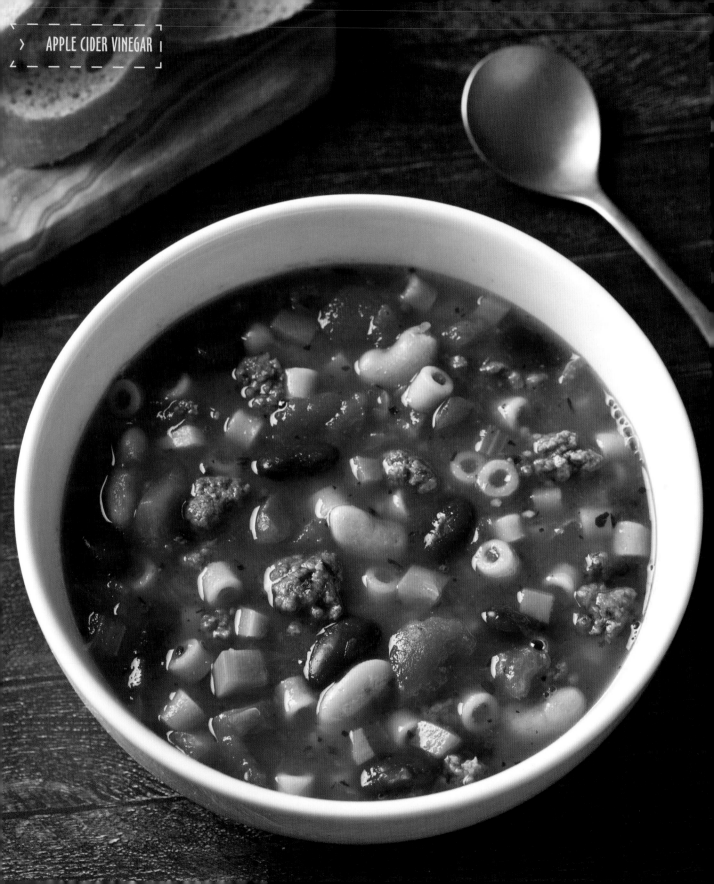

PASTA FAGIOLI
Makes 8 servings

- 2 tablespoons olive oil, divided
- 1 pound ground beef
- 1 cup chopped onion
- 1 cup diced carrots (about 2 medium)
- 1 cup diced celery (about 2 stalks)
- 3 cloves garlic, minced
- 4 cups beef broth
- 1 can (28 ounces) diced tomatoes
- 1 can (15 ounces) tomato sauce
- 1 tablespoon apple cider vinegar
- 2 teaspoons sugar
- 1½ teaspoons dried basil
- 1¼ teaspoons salt
- 1 teaspoon dried oregano
- ¾ teaspoon dried thyme
- 2 cups uncooked ditalini pasta
- 1 can (15 ounces) dark red kidney beans, rinsed and drained
- 1 can (15 ounces) cannellini beans, rinsed and drained French bread (optional)

1. Heat 1 tablespoon oil in large saucepan or Dutch oven over medium-high heat. Add beef; cook 5 minutes or until browned, stirring to break up meat. Remove to medium bowl; set aside. Drain fat from saucepan.

2. Heat remaining 1 tablespoon oil in same saucepan over medium-high heat. Add onion, carrots and celery; cook and stir 5 minutes or until vegetables are tender. Add garlic; cook and stir 1 minute. Add cooked beef, broth, tomatoes, tomato sauce, vinegar, sugar, basil, salt, oregano and thyme; bring to a boil. Reduce heat to medium-low. Cover and simmer 30 minutes.

3. Add pasta, kidney beans and cannellini beans; cook and stir over medium heat 10 minutes or until pasta is tender. Ladle into bowls. Serve with bread, if desired.

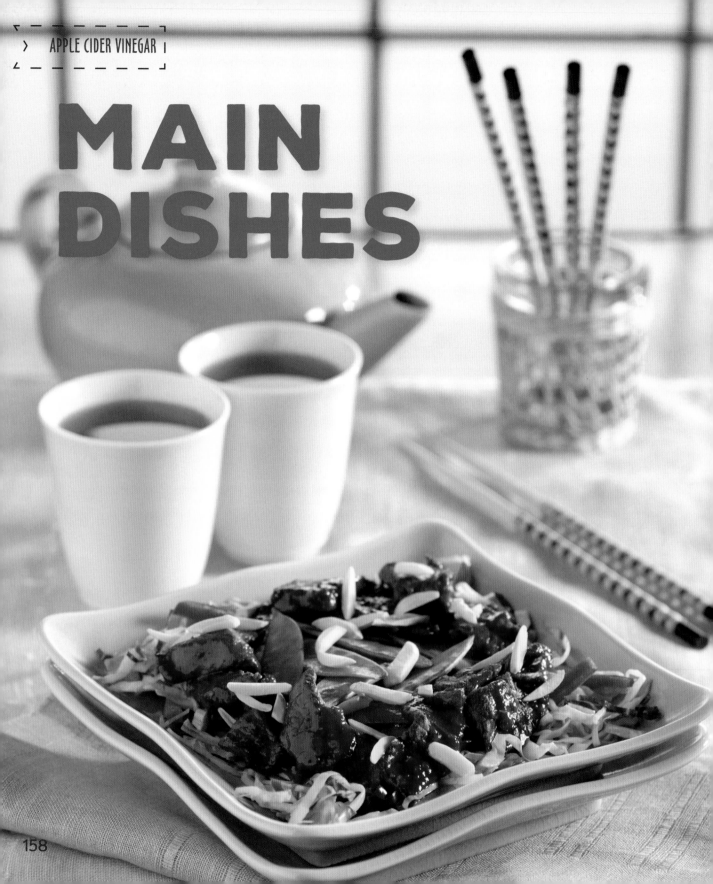

MAIN DISHES

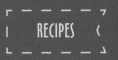

HOISIN BEEF STIR-FRY

Makes 4 servings

3   tablespoons hoisin sauce

   Grated peel and juice from 1 medium orange

1   tablespoon apple cider vinegar

⅛ to ¼ teaspoon red pepper flakes

   Nonstick cooking spray

1½ cups (3 ounces) snow peas

1   medium red bell pepper, cut into strips

½   teaspoon dark sesame oil

4   cups packaged coleslaw mix or shredded cabbage

¼   teaspoon salt

12 ounces sirloin steak, cut into thin strips

¼   cup (1 ounce) slivered almonds, toasted*

1. Combine hoisin sauce, orange peel and juice, vinegar and red pepper flakes in small bowl; stir to blend. Set aside.

2. Spray large skillet with cooking spray. Add snow peas, bell peppers and sesame oil; cook and stir 2 minutes. Add coleslaw and salt; cook and stir 2 minutes. Remove to large serving dish; keep warm.

3. Add steak to same skillet; cook and stir 2 minutes. Arrange with vegetables; keep warm.

4. Add hoisin mixture to skillet; cook and stir 2 minutes or until sauce reduces to ¼ cup. Spoon over steak. Sprinkle with almonds.

*To toast almonds, cook and stir in small skillet over medium heat 1 to 2 minutes or until lightly browned.

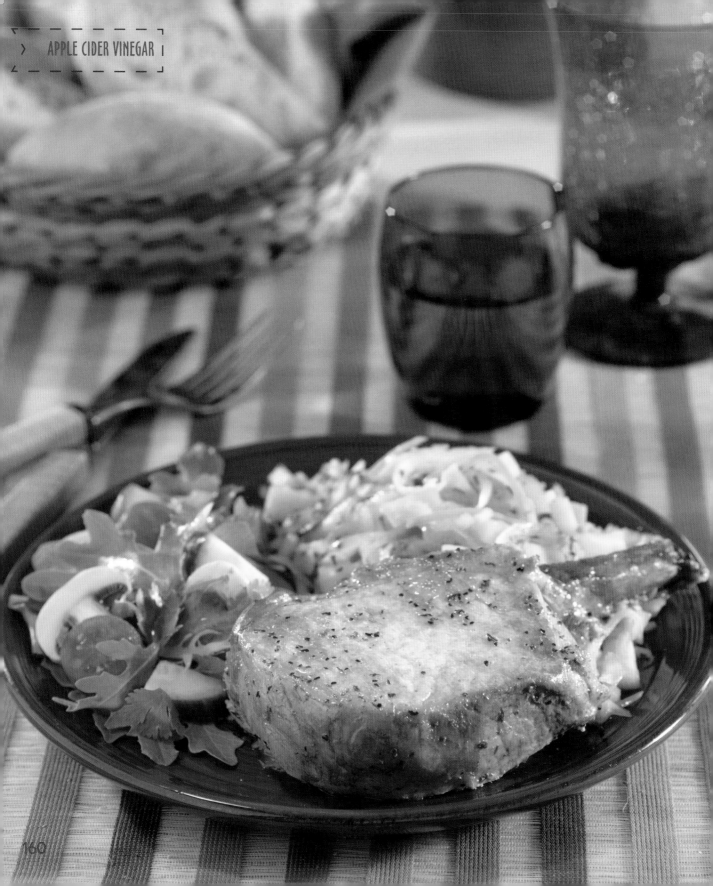

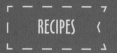

ROASTED PORK CHOPS WITH APPLE AND CABBAGE
Makes 4 servings

- 3 teaspoons olive oil, divided
- ½ medium onion, thinly sliced
- 2 cloves garlic, minced
- 1 teaspoon dried thyme
- 4 bone-in pork chops (6 to 8 ounces each), cut about 1 inch thick
  Salt and black pepper
- ¼ cup apple cider vinegar
- 1 tablespoon packed brown sugar
- 1 large McIntosh apple, peeled and chopped
- ½ (8-ounce) package shredded coleslaw mix

1. Preheat oven to 375°F.

2. Heat 2 teaspoons oil in large ovenproof skillet over medium-high heat. Add onion; cook and stir 4 to 6 minutes or until tender. Add garlic and thyme; cook and stir 30 seconds. Remove to small bowl.

3. Heat remaining 1 teaspoon oil in same skillet. Season pork chops with salt and pepper. Add to skillet; cook 2 minutes per side or until browned. Remove pork chops from skillet.

4. Remove skillet from heat. Add vinegar, brown sugar and ¼ teaspoon pepper; stir to dissolve sugar and scrape up browned bits from bottom of skillet. Add onion mixture, apple and coleslaw mix. *Do not stir.*

5. Arrange pork chops on top of cabbage mixture, overlapping to fit. Cover; bake 15 minutes or until pork chops are barely pink in center.

TIP: This recipe can be made up to a day ahead. Prepare and separately wrap pork chops and cabbage-apple mixture. Refrigerate until ready to serve. Preheat oven to 375°F. Place cabbage mixture in large ovenproof skillet. Heat over medium-high heat. Cook and stir until blended and liquid comes to a boil. Lay pork chops on top of cabbage mixture, overlapping to fit. Continue as directed in recipe.

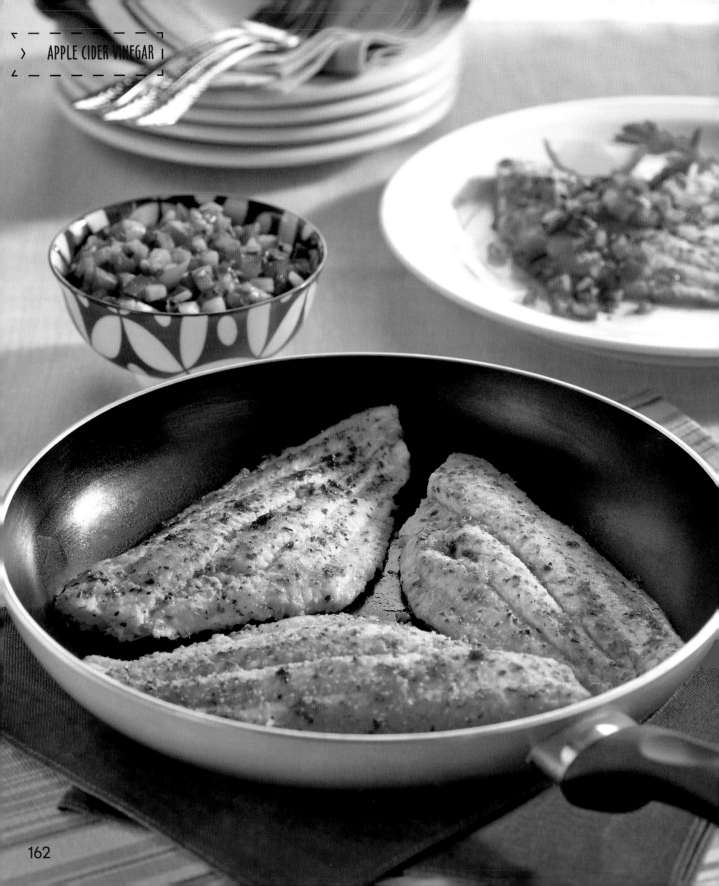

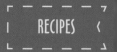

SKILLET-GRILLED CATFISH AND CREOLE SALSA

Makes 4 servings

- 4 catfish fillets (4 ounces each), rinsed and patted dry
- 1 teaspoon steak seasoning or blackened seasoning
- ½ teaspoon salt, divided
- 1 cup finely chopped tomatoes
- ⅓ cup finely chopped green bell pepper
- ¼ cup finely chopped celery
- ¼ cup minced green onions (white and green parts)
- 2 tablespoons minced fresh parsley
- 2 teaspoons apple cider vinegar
- ¼ teaspoon dried thyme
- ¼ to ½ teaspoon hot pepper sauce
  Nonstick cooking spray
- 4 lemon wedges

1. Sprinkle one side of each fillet evenly with steak seasoning and ¼ teaspoon salt. Combine tomatoes, bell pepper, celery, green onions, parsley, vinegar, thyme, remaining ¼ teaspoon salt and hot pepper sauce in medium bowl; stir to blend. Set aside.

2. Spray large skillet with cooking spray; heat over medium-high heat. Add fillets, seasoned side down; cook 3 minutes. Turn; cook 3 minutes or until fillets are opaque in center. Squeeze lemon wedges over all. Serve with salsa.

SERVING SUGGESTIONS: Serve with quick-cooking brown rice and/or coleslaw.

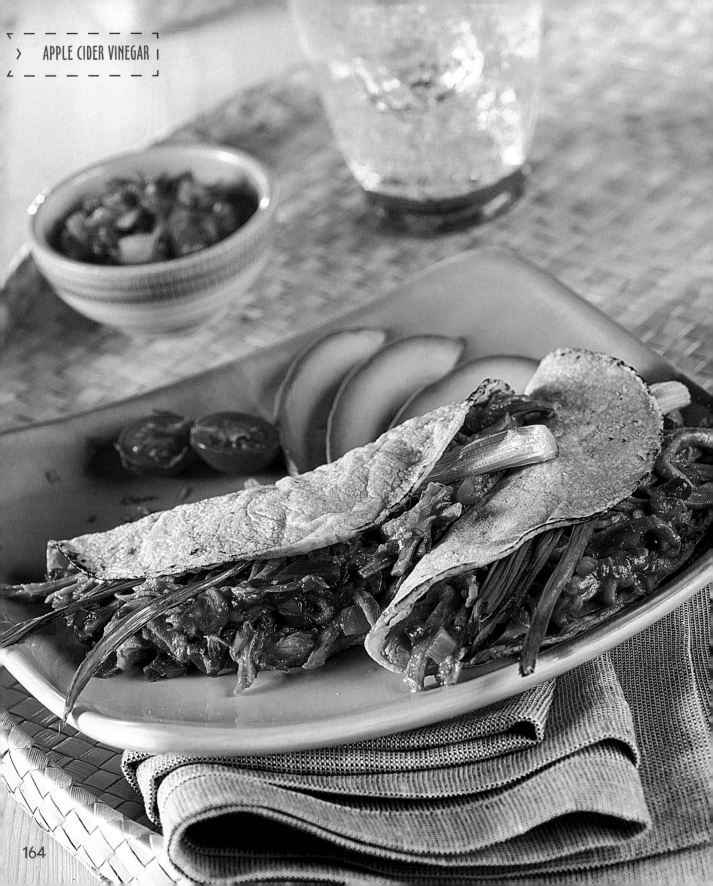

SHREDDED CHIPOTLE PORK TACOS WITH ROASTED GREEN ONIONS

Makes 16 tacos

6	cups water
2	pounds boneless pork shoulder, cut into 2-inch pieces
1	medium onion, thinly sliced
4	tablespoons apple cider vinegar, divided
1	teaspoon salt
1	tablespoon olive oil
1	cup finely chopped onion
4	cloves garlic, minced
1	can (about 8 ounces) tomato sauce
3	chipotle peppers in adobo sauce, finely chopped and mashed with a fork
½	teaspoon ground cumin
16	(6-inch) corn tortillas, warmed
	Roasted Green Onions (recipe follows)
	Salt

1. Bring water to a boil in Dutch oven over high heat. Add pork, sliced onion, 3 tablespoons vinegar and salt; return to a boil. Reduce heat; simmer, partially covered, 1½ hours. Remove pork with slotted spoon and cool slightly; reserve 1 cup cooking liquid. Remove pork to large cutting board; shred using two forks.

2. Heat oil in large skillet over medium-high heat. Add chopped onion; cook and stir 3 minutes. Add garlic; cook 15 seconds. Add tomato sauce, chipotle peppers, cumin, remaining 1 tablespoon vinegar, shredded pork and reserved cooking liquid; cook and stir 2 minutes until heated through. Remove from heat; cover and let stand 10 minutes.

3. Fill each tortilla evenly with pork mixture and Roasted Green Onions.

ROASTED GREEN ONIONS: Preheat oven to 425°F. Trim 16 green onions; place on large baking sheet. Drizzle with 2 teaspoons olive oil; toss gently to coat. Arrange in single layer and bake 10 minutes. Sprinkle with salt.

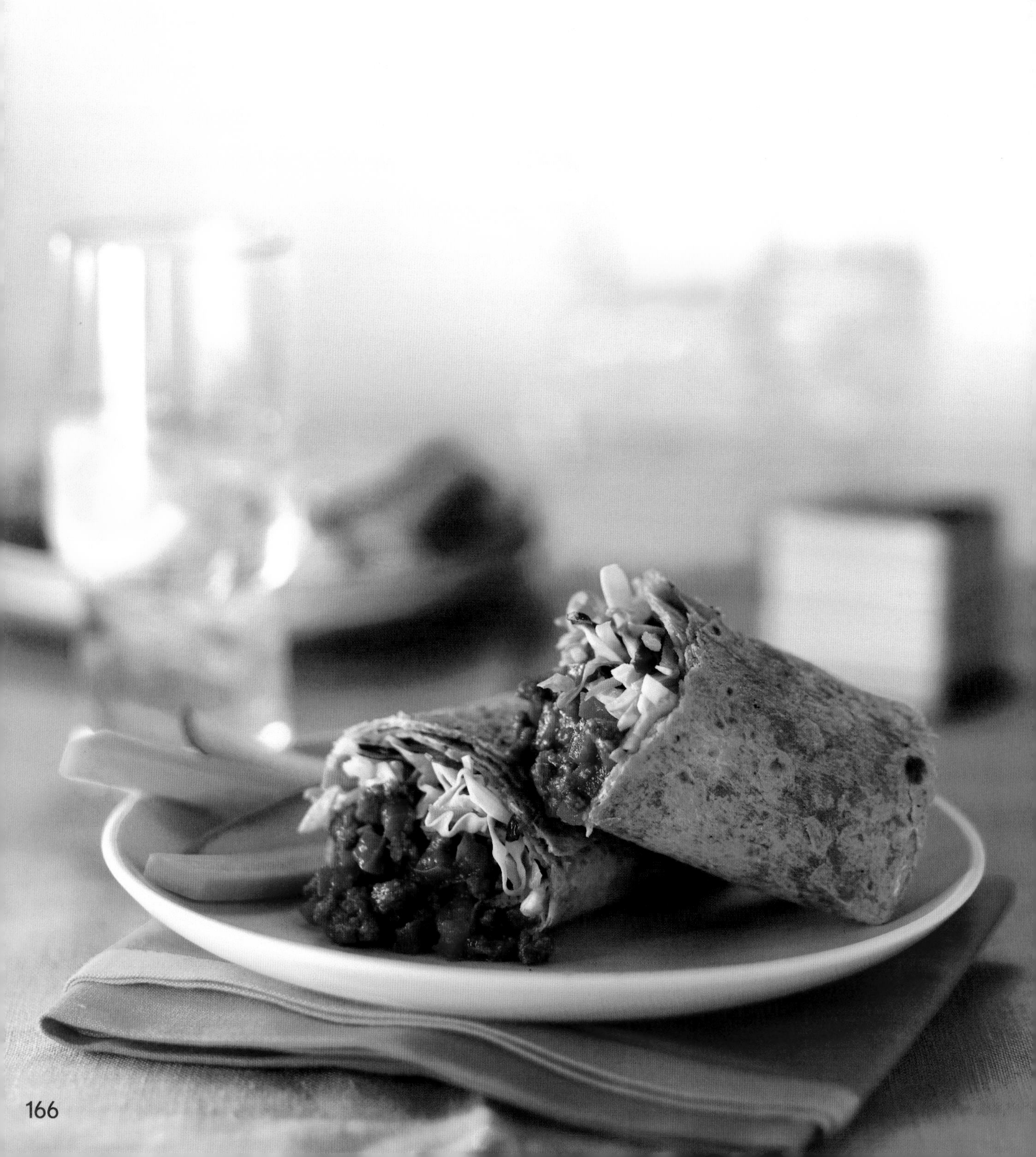

SLOPPY JOE BURRITOS
Makes 4 servings

~~~~~~~~~~~~~~~~~~~~~~~~~~~~~~~~~~~~~~

- 1   tablespoon apple cider vinegar
- 1   teaspoon sugar
- 1   teaspoon vegetable oil
- ¼   teaspoon salt
- 2   cups coleslaw mix
- 1   pound ground beef
- 1   cup *each* chopped red and green bell peppers
- ½   cup chopped onion
- 1   can (about 16 ounces) sloppy joe sauce
- 4   (7- to 8-inch) colored tortilla wraps

1. Whisk vinegar, sugar, oil and salt in medium bowl until well blended. Add coleslaw mix; toss to coat. Set aside.

2. Brown beef in large skillet over medium-high heat 6 to 8 minutes, stirring to break up meat. Drain fat. Stir in sloppy joe sauce; cook 3 minutes or until slightly thickened and heated through.

3. Add bell peppers and onion; cook and stir 4 to 6 minutes or until vegetables are tender.

4. Divide meat mixture evenly among tortillas. Top each with ½ cup coleslaw mixture. Roll up tortillas, folding in sides to enclose filling.

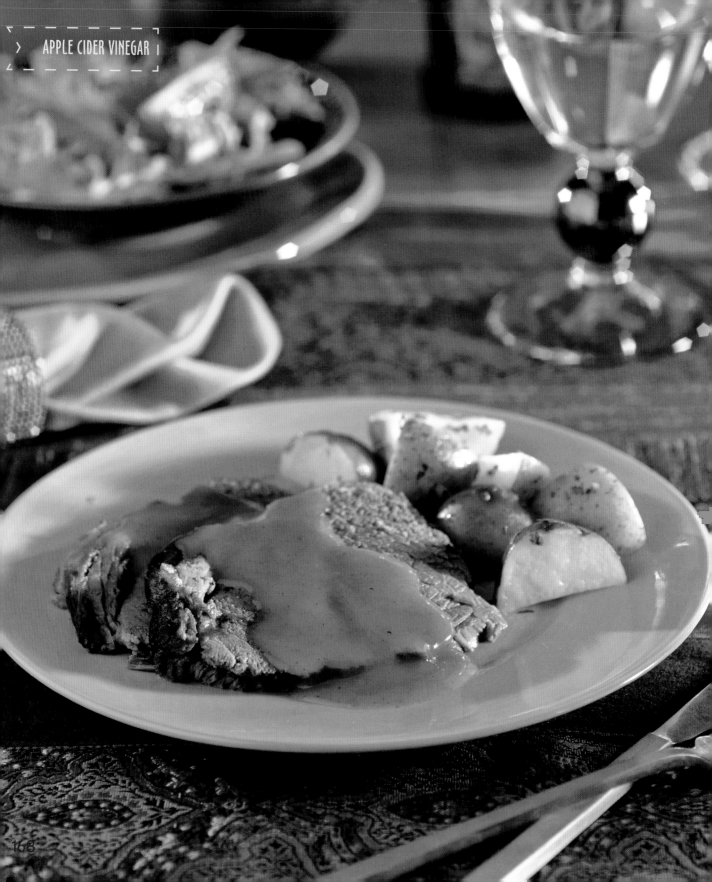

SAUERBRATEN WITH GINGERSNAP GRAVY

Makes 6 to 8 servings

3 cups water

1 cup apple cider vinegar

1 onion, thinly sliced

3 tablespoons brown sugar

2 cloves garlic, crushed

1½ teaspoons salt

1 teaspoon ground ginger

1 teaspoon whole allspice

1 teaspoon whole cloves

½ teaspoon juniper berries

1 beef rump roast (about 4 pounds)

2 tablespoons vegetable oil

2 tablespoons all-purpose flour

¼ cup crushed gingersnaps

1. Combine water and vinegar in large saucepan; bring to a boil over high heat. Remove from heat. Stir in onion, brown sugar, garlic, salt, ginger, allspice, cloves and juniper berries; cool slightly.

2. Place roast in large resealable food storage bag. Pour marinade over roast; seal bag. Marinate in refrigerator at least 8 hours or overnight, turning occasionally.

3. Remove roast from marinade, reserving marinade. Pat roast dry with paper towels. Heat oil in Dutch oven over medium-high heat. Brown roast 6 to 8 minutes on all sides. Add marinade to Dutch oven. Reduce heat to low. Cover; cook 2½ to 3¼ hours or until fork-tender. Remove roast from Dutch oven; set aside.

4. Strain braising liquid through fine mesh sieve into large bowl; discard spices and onion. Skim fat from braising liquid; discard. Measure 2 cups braising liquid; discard remaining liquid. Place 1½ cups liquid in Dutch oven. Stir ½ cup liquid into flour in small bowl; whisk into liquid in Dutch oven. Add gingersnaps; mix well. Bring to a boil over high heat.

5. Return roast to Dutch oven. Reduce heat to low. Cover; cook 15 to 20 minutes until flavors blend and sauce thickens. Slice roast and serve with sauce.

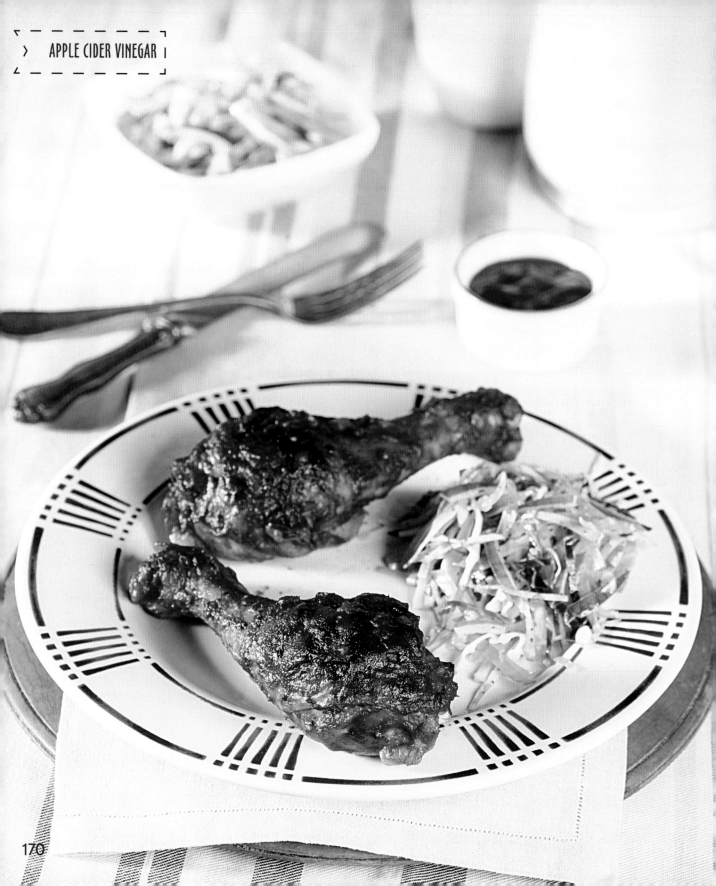

OVEN-BARBECUED CHICKEN
Makes 8 to 10 servings

2	tablespoons vegetable oil, divided
1	large onion, chopped
1/3	cup dark brown sugar
1/3	cup apple cider vinegar
1	can (28 ounces) tomato purée
2	teaspoons chili powder
1	teaspoon mustard powder
1¼	teaspoons salt, divided
1	teaspoon freshly ground black pepper, divided
¼	teaspoon liquid smoke
1	(6- to 7-pound) chicken, cut into 8 pieces (about 5 pounds chicken pieces)

1. Heat 1 tablespoon oil in medium saucepan over medium-high heat. Add onion; cook 5 minutes or until softened. Add brown sugar and vinegar, stir to blend. Add tomato purée, chili powder, mustard powder, 1 teaspoon salt, $3/4$ teaspoon pepper and liquid smoke; stir to blend. Bring mixture to a boil over high heat. Reduce heat to low. Simmer 45 minutes or until mixture thickens slightly, stirring occasionally.

2. Meanwhile, move rack to middle of oven. Preheat oven to 450°F. Place chicken pieces on large baking sheet. Brush chicken with remaining 1 tablespoon oil and season with remaining $1/4$ teaspoon salt and $1/4$ teaspoon pepper.

3. Bake chicken 35 minutes or until internal temperature of thighs is 160°F. Transfer rack to upper part of oven. Dollop sauce over chicken pieces; spread evenly with back of spoon. Broil 10 minutes 6 inches from heating element until bubbly and beginning to brown. Serve warm.

TIP: As the sauce thickens, keep the heat low to keep spattering to a minimum, for both safety and ease in cleaning up. Refrigerate any extra sauce for later use.

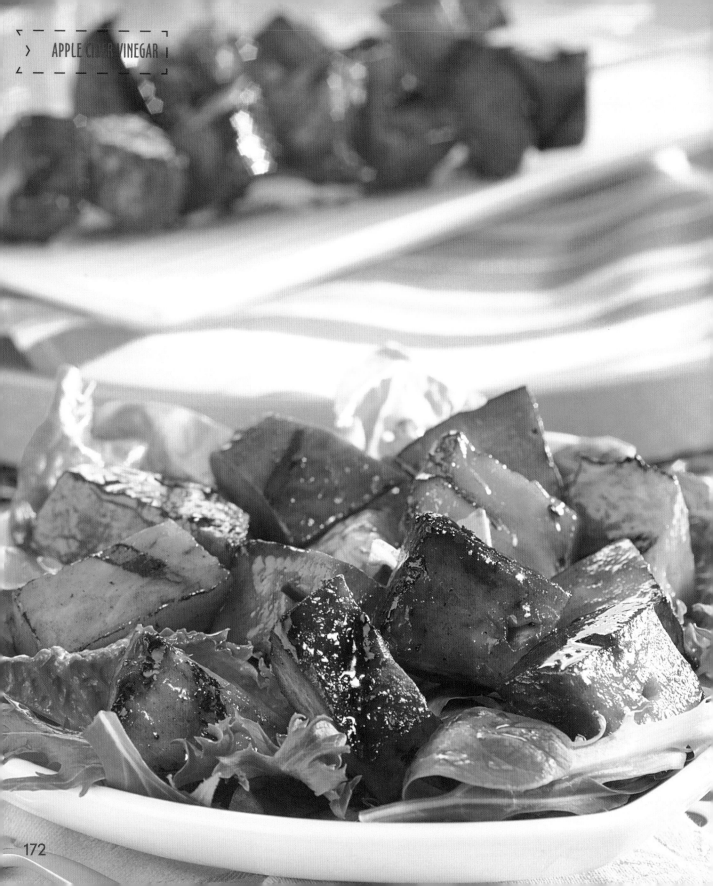

GLAZED HAM AND SWEET POTATO KABOBS
Makes 4 servings

- 1 sweet potato (about 12 ounces), peeled
- 1/4 cup water
- 1/4 cup (1/2 stick) butter
- 1/4 cup packed dark brown sugar
- 2 tablespoons apple cider vinegar
- 2 tablespoons molasses
- 1 tablespoon yellow mustard
- 1 tablespoon Worcestershire sauce
- 3/4 teaspoon ground cinnamon
- 1/2 teaspoon ground allspice
- 1/8 teaspoon red pepper flakes
- 1 boneless ham slice (about 12 ounces),
  1/4 inch thick, cut into 20 (1-inch) pieces
- 16 fresh pineapple chunks (about 1 inch)
- 1 package (10 ounces) mixed salad greens

1. Soak 4 (12-inch) wooden skewers in water 20 minutes.

2. Meanwhile, cut sweet potato into 16 pieces; place in shallow microwavable dish with water. Cover; microwave on HIGH 4 minutes or until fork-tender. Drain. Spread potatoes in single layer; cool 5 minutes.

3. Combine butter, brown sugar, vinegar, molasses, mustard, Worcestershire sauce, cinnamon, allspice and red pepper flakes in medium saucepan; bring to a boil over medium-high heat. Cook 2 minutes or until reduced to 1/2 cup. Remove from heat; cool slightly.

4. Prepare grill for direct cooking. Oil grid. Alternately thread ham, sweet potato and pineapple onto skewers, beginning and ending with ham. Grill skewers over medium heat 6 to 8 minutes or until sweet potato is browned and ham is heated through, turning every 2 minutes and brushing with glaze. Cover; let stand 5 minutes. Remove ham, sweet potato and pineapple from skewers; serve over greens.

VARIATION: Toast 6 to 8 large marshmallows on skewers alongside the kabobs. Separate the sweet potatoes and top with warm marshmallows.

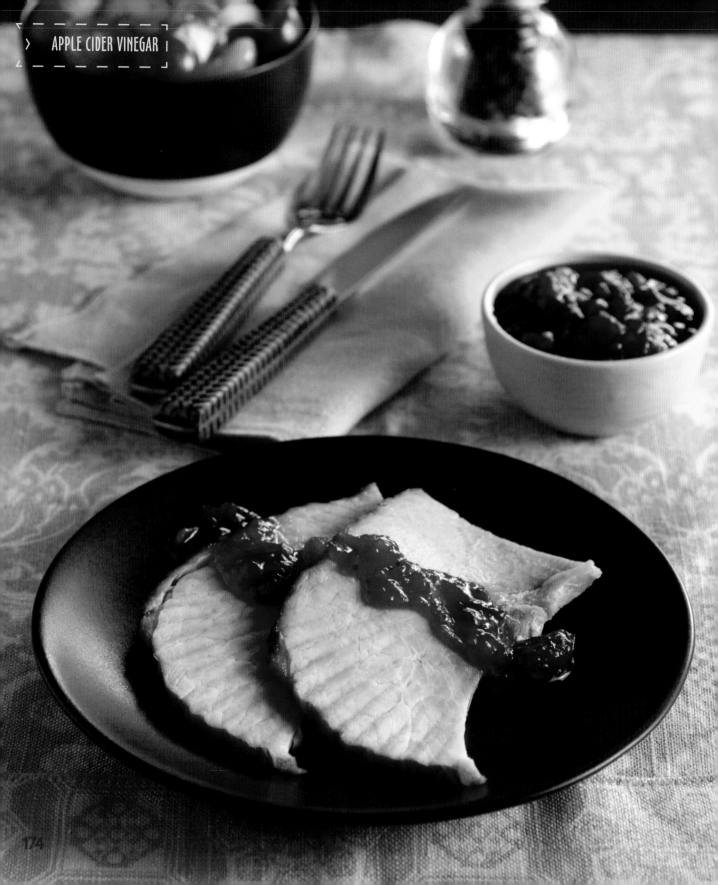

HONEY GLAZED HAM WITH CRANBERRY CHUTNEY
Makes 32 servings

1 (9-pound) bone-in, fully cooked, spiral-cut smoked ham half

¼ cup honey

1 tablespoon water

½ teaspoon Dijon mustard

1 teaspoon olive oil

3 shallots, chopped

1 tablespoon minced peeled fresh ginger

2 cans (14 ounces each) whole berry cranberry sauce

¼ cup apple cider vinegar

⅛ to ¼ teaspoon salt

1. Preheat oven to 350°F. Unwrap ham; trim fat. Place face down on large baking dish coated with nonstick cooking spray; cover loosely with foil. Bake 1 hour and 45 minutes.

2. Meanwhile, combine honey, water and mustard in medium bowl; stir to blend. Set aside.

3. Heat oil in large skillet over medium-high heat. Add shallots and ginger; cook 3 minutes or until shallots become soft. Stir in cranberry sauce, vinegar and salt; cook 2 minutes, stirring occasionally. Remove from heat. Let stand 2 hours.

4. To serve, remove foil from ham; brush with honey glaze. Bake, uncovered, 15 minutes or until internal temperature is 140°F. Serve with Cranberry Chutney.

175

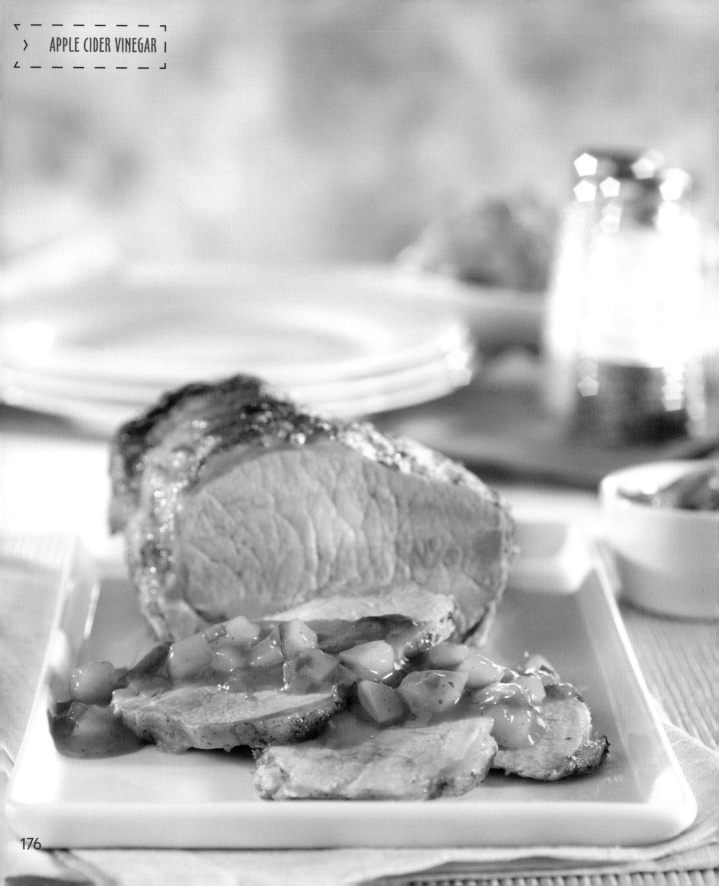

ROASTED PORK LOIN IN CHILI-SPICE SAUCE

Makes 6 servings

- 1 cup chopped onion
- ¼ cup orange juice
- 2 cloves garlic
- 1 tablespoon apple cider vinegar
- 1½ teaspoons chili powder
- ¼ teaspoon dried thyme
- ¼ teaspoon ground cumin
- ¼ teaspoon ground cinnamon
- ⅛ teaspoon ground allspice
- ⅛ teaspoon ground cloves
- 1½ pounds pork loin, fat trimmed
- 3 firm large bananas
- 2 limes
- 1 ripe large papaya, peeled, seeded and cubed
- 1 green onion, minced

1. Preheat oven to 350°F. Combine onion, orange juice and garlic in food processor or blender; process until finely chopped. Pour into medium saucepan. Stir in vinegar, chili powder, thyme, cumin, cinnamon, allspice and cloves; simmer over medium-high heat about 5 minutes or until thickened. Cut ¼-inch-deep lengthwise slits down top and bottom of roast at 1½-inch intervals. Spread about 1 tablespoon spice paste over bottom; place roast in baking pan. Spread remaining 2 tablespoons spice paste over sides and top, working mixture into slits; cover with foil. Bake 45 minutes or until meat thermometer registers 140°F.

2. Remove roast from oven. *Increase oven temperature to 450°F.* Pour off liquid; discard. Return roast to oven. Bake, uncovered, 15 minutes or until spice mixture browns lightly and meat thermometer registers 150°F in center of roast. Remove from oven; tent with foil and let stand 5 minutes before slicing.

3. Meanwhile, spray 9-inch pie plate or cake pan with nonstick cooking spray. Peel bananas and slice diagonally into ½-inch-thick pieces. Place in prepared pan. Squeeze juice from 1 lime over bananas; toss to coat. Cover; bake 5 minutes or until heated through. Stir in papaya, juice of remaining lime and green onion. Serve with roast.

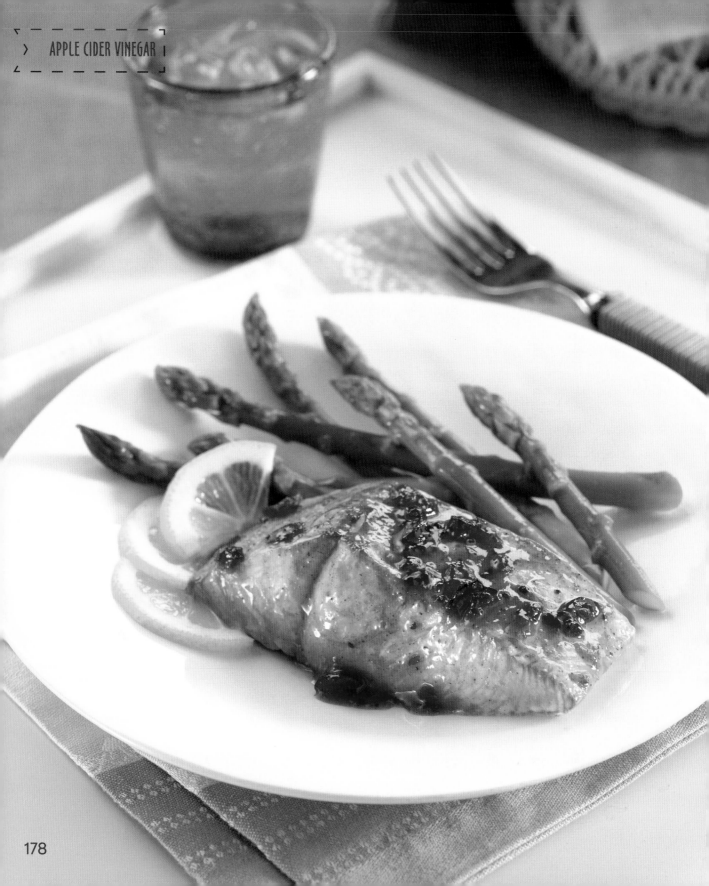

CRANBERRY CHUTNEY GLAZED SALMON
Makes 4 servings

~~~~~~~~~~~~~~~~~~~~~~~~~~~~~~~~~~

½   teaspoon salt

½   teaspoon ground cinnamon

¼   teaspoon ground red pepper

4   skinless salmon fillets (5 to 6 ounces each)

¼   cup cranberry chutney

1   tablespoon apple cider vinegar

1. Preheat broiler or prepare grill for indirect cooking. Combine salt, cinnamon and ground red pepper in small cup; sprinkle over salmon. Combine chutney and vinegar in small bowl; brush small amount evenly over each salmon fillet.

2. Broil 5 to 6 inches from heat source or grill over medium-hot coals on covered grill 4 to 6 minutes or until salmon is opaque in center.

VARIATION: If cranberry chutney is not available, substitute mango chutney. Chop any large pieces of mango.

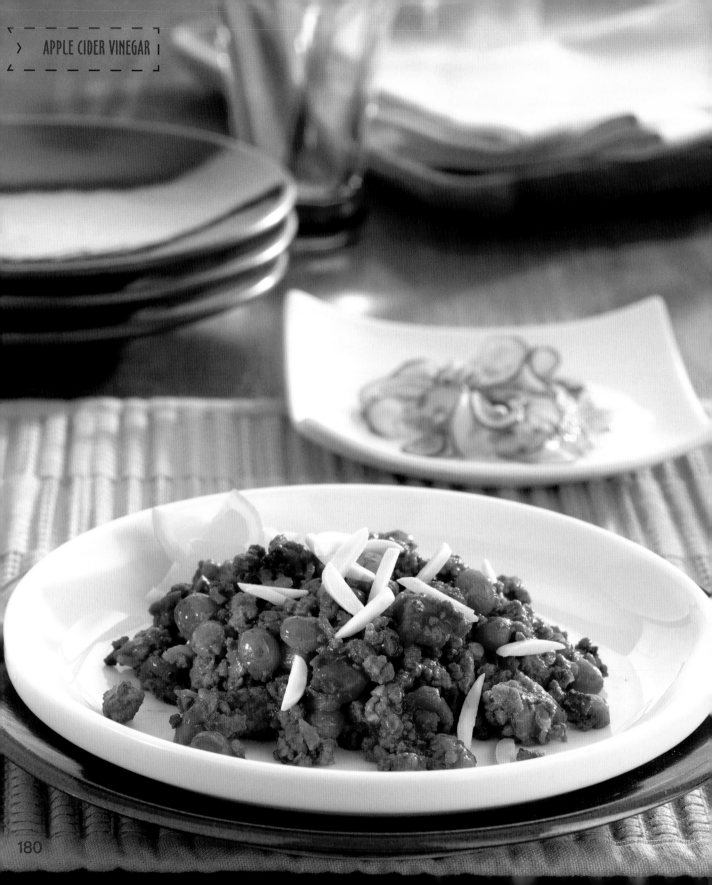

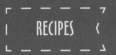

PICADILLO

Makes 4 servings

- 1   pound ground beef
- 1   small onion, chopped
- 1   clove garlic, minced
- 1   can (14½ ounces) diced tomatoes, undrained
- ¼   cup golden raisins
- 1   tablespoon chili powder
- 1   tablespoon apple cider vinegar
- ½   teaspoon ground cumin
- ½   teaspoon dried oregano
- ½   teaspoon ground cinnamon
- ¼   teaspoon red pepper flakes
- 1   teaspoon salt
- ¼   cup slivered almonds (optional)

SLOW COOKER DIRECTIONS

1. Brown ground beef, onion and garlic in large nonstick skillet over medium heat 6 to 8 minutes, stirring to break up meat; drain fat. Remove mixture to slow cooker.

2. Add tomatoes, raisins, chili powder, vinegar, cumin, oregano, cinnamon and red pepper flakes to slow cooker. Cover; cook on LOW 6 to 7 hours. Stir in salt. Garnish with almonds.

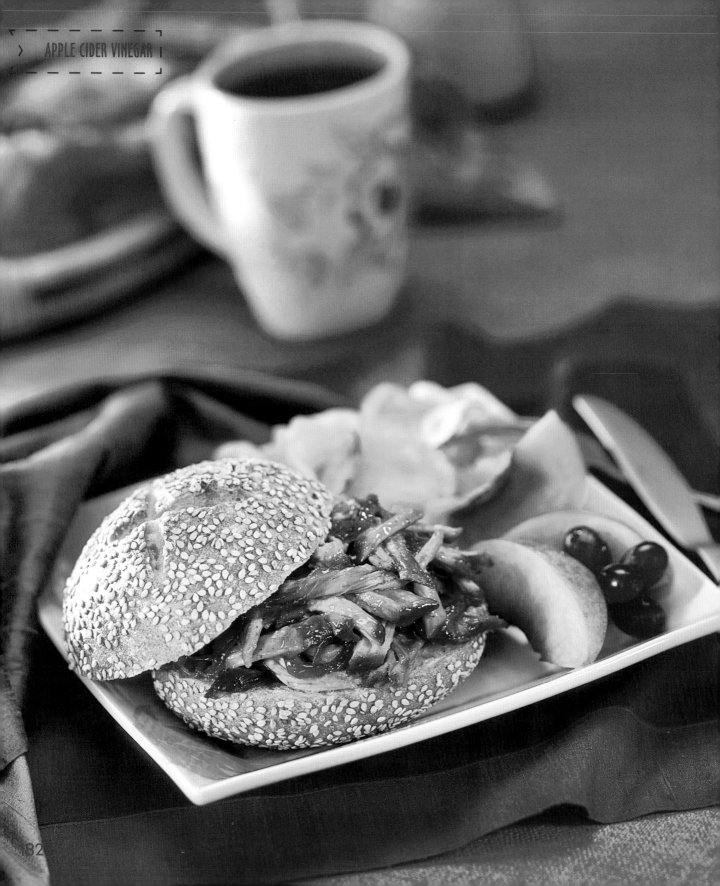

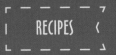

SHREDDED APRICOT PORK SANDWICHES
Makes 10 to 12 sandwiches

- 2 medium onions, thinly sliced
- 1 cup apricot preserves
- ½ cup packed dark brown sugar
- ½ cup barbecue sauce
- ¼ cup apple cider vinegar
- 2 tablespoons Worcestershire sauce
- ½ teaspoon red pepper flakes
- 1 (4-pound) boneless pork top loin roast, trimmed of fat
- ¼ cup cold water
- 2 tablespoons cornstarch
- 1 tablespoon grated fresh ginger
  Salt and black pepper
- 10 to 12 sesame or onion rolls, toasted

SLOW COOKER DIRECTIONS

1. Combine onions, preserves, brown sugar, barbecue sauce, vinegar, Worcestershire sauce and red pepper flakes in small bowl; stir to blend. Place pork roast in 5-quart slow cooker. Pour apricot mixture over roast; turn to coat. Cover; cook on LOW 8 to 9 hours.

2. Remove pork to large cutting board; shred pork using two forks. Let cooking liquid stand 5 minutes to allow fat to rise. Skim fat.

3. *Turn slow cooker to HIGH.* Combine water, cornstarch, ginger, salt and pepper in small bowl until smooth; whisk into cooking liquid. Cover; cook on HIGH 10 to 15 or until thickened. Return shredded pork to slow cooker; mix well. Serve on toasted rolls.

VARIATION: A 4-pound pork shoulder roast, cut into pieces and trimmed of fat, can be substituted for the pork loin roast.

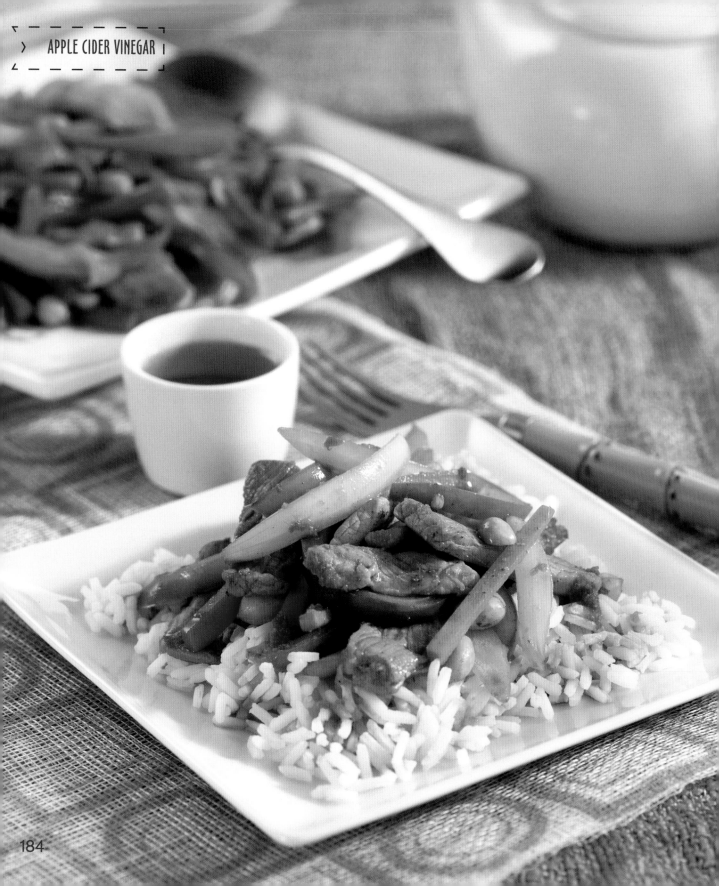

PORK AND TOASTED PEANUT TOSS
Makes 4 servings

- 3 tablespoons soy sauce
- 3 tablespoons apple cider vinegar
- 2 tablespoons water
- 2 tablespoons plus 2 teaspoons sugar
- 2 teaspoons grated fresh ginger
- ⅛ teaspoon salt
- ⅛ teaspoon red pepper flakes
  Nonstick cooking spray
- ½ pound pork tenderloin, cut into thin strips
- 1 medium onion, cut into 8 wedges
- 1 large green bell pepper, thinly sliced
- 1 medium carrot, cut into thin strips
- ¼ cup plus 2 tablespoons dry-roasted peanuts
  Hot cooked rice

1. Combine soy sauce, vinegar, water, sugar, ginger, salt and red pepper flakes in small saucepan; stir to blend. Heat over medium heat until heated through.

2. Meanwhile, spray large skillet with cooking spray. Add pork; cook and stir 3 minutes or until no longer pink. Add onion, bell pepper, carrot and peanuts; cook and stir 4 minutes or until crisp-tender. Serve pork mixture over rice; top with sauce.

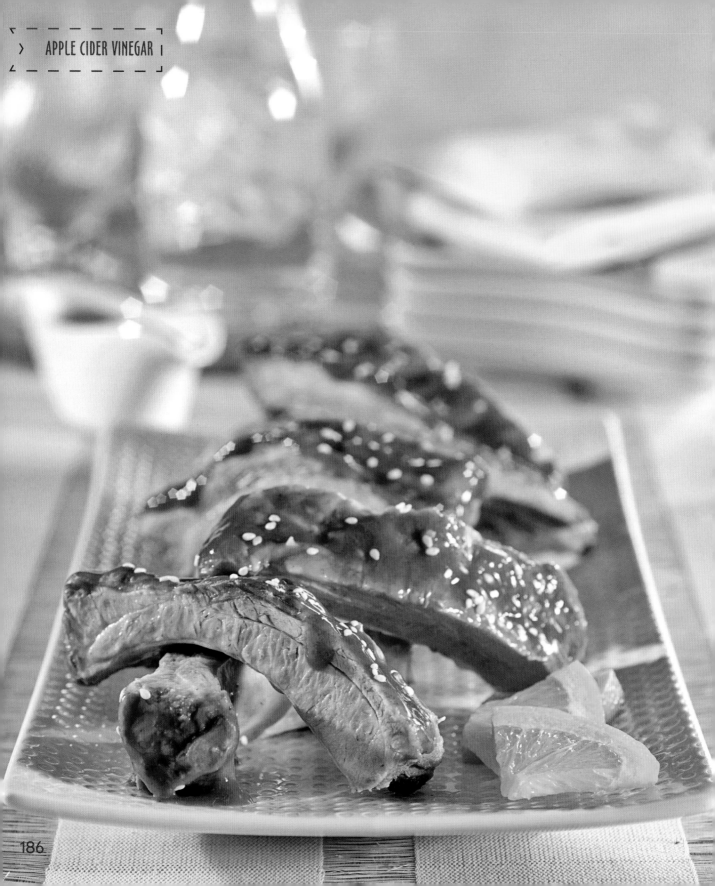

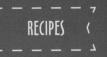
HONEY GINGER RIBS

Makes about 4 servings

¼ cup plus 1 tablespoon soy sauce, divided

3 tablespoons hoisin sauce

3 tablespoons dry sherry, divided

1 tablespoon sugar

1 teaspoon minced fresh ginger

2 cloves garlic, minced

¼ teaspoon Chinese five-spice powder**

1 rack pork spareribs* (about 2 pounds), cut into 6-inch pieces and fat trimmed

2 tablespoons honey

1 tablespoon apple cider vinegar

Sesame seeds (optional)

*Ask your butcher to cut ribs down length of rack into two pieces so that each half is 2 to 3 inches wide.

**Chinese five-spice powder consists of cinnamon, cloves, fennel seed, star anise and Szechuan peppercorns. It can be found at Asian markets and in most supermarkets.

1. Combine ¼ cup soy sauce, hoisin sauce, 2 table-spoons sherry, sugar, ginger, garlic and five-spice powder in large resealable food storage bag; add ribs. Seal bag. Refrigerate 8 hours or overnight, turning bag occasionally.

2. Preheat oven to 350°F. Line large baking sheet with foil. Place ribs on rack in pan, reserving mari-nade. Bake 30 minutes; turn over. Brush with mari-nade; bake 40 minutes or until ribs are tender when pierced with fork.

3. Combine honey, vinegar, remaining 1 tablespoon soy sauce and 1 tablespoon sherry in small bowl; mix well. Brush ½ of mixture over ribs. Place under broiler 4 to 6 inches from heat source; broil 2 to 3 minutes or until ribs are glazed. Turn ribs over. Brush with remaining honey mixture. Broil 2 to 3 minutes or until glazed. Cut into individual pieces. Sprinkle with sesame seeds, if desired.

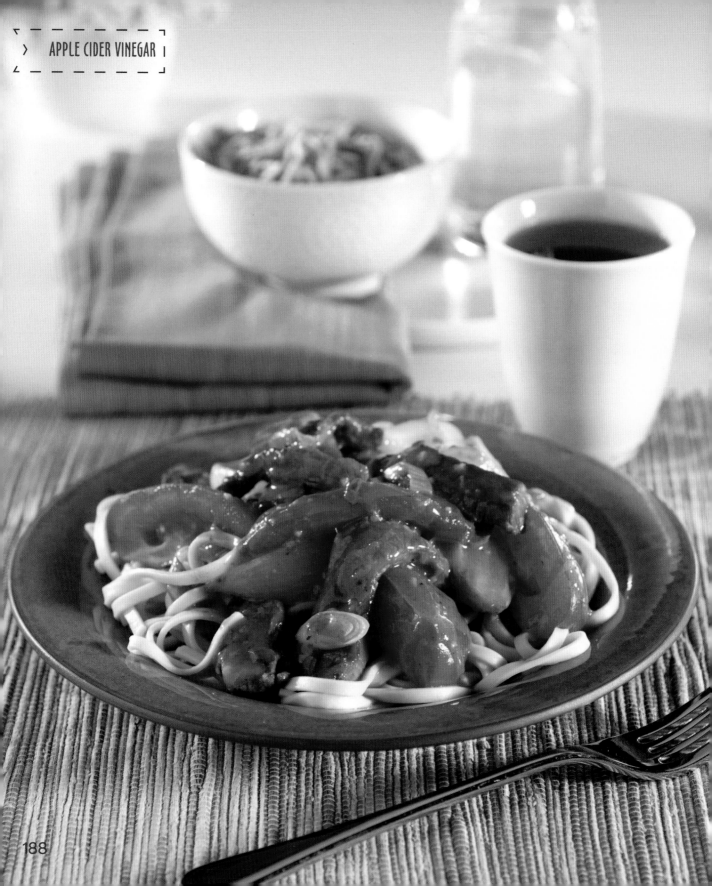

CANTONESE TOMATO BEEF

Makes 4 servings

- 1 beef flank steak (about 1 pound)
- 2 tablespoons soy sauce
- 2 tablespoons dark sesame oil, divided
- 1 tablespoon plus 1 teaspoon cornstarch, divided
- 1 pound Chinese-style thin wheat noodles
- 1 cup beef broth
- 2 tablespoons packed brown sugar
- 1 tablespoon apple cider vinegar
- 2 tablespoons vegetable oil, divided
- 1 tablespoon minced fresh ginger
- 3 small onions, cut into wedges
- 2 pounds ripe tomatoes (5 large), cored and cut into wedges
- 1 green onion, diagonally cut into thin slices

1. Cut flank steak lengthwise in half, then crosswise into 1/4-inch-thick slices. Combine soy sauce, 1 tablespoon sesame oil and 1 teaspoon cornstarch in large bowl. Add beef slices; toss to coat. Set aside.

2. Cook noodles according to package directions. Drain; toss with remaining 1 tablespoon sesame oil. Keep warm. Combine broth, brown sugar, remaining 1 tablespoon cornstarch and vinegar in small bowl; set aside.

3. Heat 1 tablespoon oil in large skillet over high heat 1 minute. Add beef and marinade; cook and stir 5 minutes or until lightly browned. Remove beef to large plate; set aside. Reduce heat to medium. Add ginger; cook and stir 30 seconds.

4. Add remaining 1 tablespoon vegetable oil to skillet. Add onion wedges; cook and stir 2 minutes. Stir in half of tomato wedges. Add broth mixture to skillet; cook and stir 5 to 8 minutes or until liquid boils and thickens.

5. Return beef and any juices to large skillet. Add remaining tomato wedges; cook and stir until heated through. Serve over noodles.

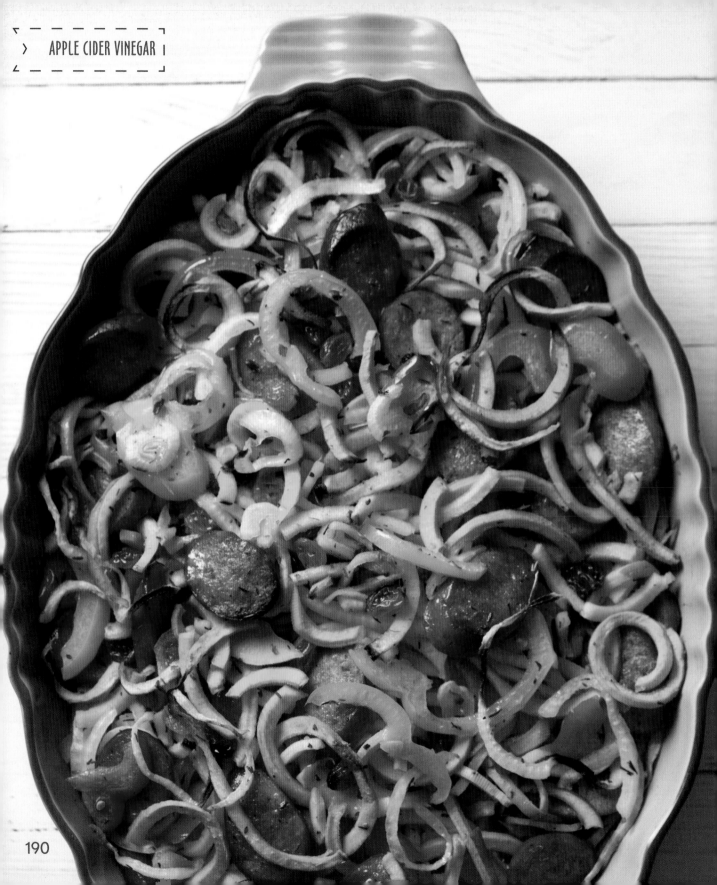

SAUSAGE, POTATO AND APPLE BAKE
Makes 6 servings

3 tablespoons packed brown sugar

1 tablespoon dried thyme

1 tablespoon dried oregano

¼ cup plus 2 tablespoons apple cider vinegar

2 sweet potatoes (1½ to 2 pounds), peeled

2 apples, such as Fuji or McIntosh, peeled

1 white onion

1 red bell pepper

1 yellow bell pepper

½ cup golden raisins

1½ pounds smoked sausage, such as kielbasa or Polish sausage, sliced diagonally into ¼-inch pieces

1. Preheat oven to 450°F. Spray 13X9-inch baking dish or 2-quart casserole with nonstick cooking spray. Combine brown sugar, thyme and oregano in large bowl; stir in vinegar until brown sugar is dissolved.

2. Spiral sweet potatoes, apples and onion with thick spiral blade. Spiral bell peppers with spiral slicing blade. Cut vegetables into desired lengths. Add vegetables and raisins to brown sugar mixture; toss to coat.

3. Remove vegetables to prepared baking dish using tongs or slotted spoon. Mix in sausage; drizzle with remaining brown sugar mixture. Bake 20 minutes or until vegetables are tender.

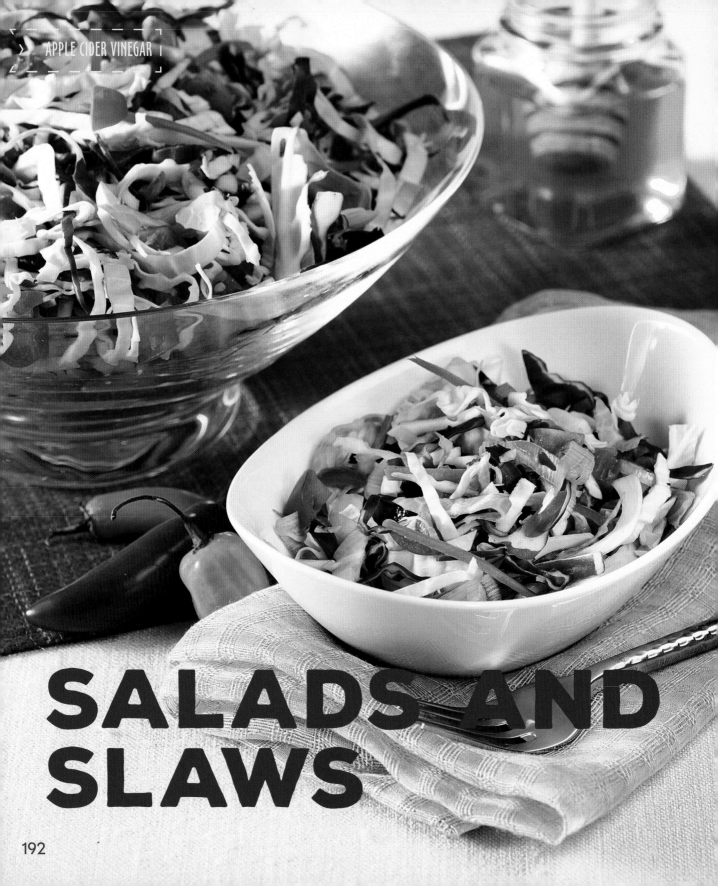

SALADS AND SLAWS

JALAPEÑO COLESLAW

Makes 8 servings

6 cups shredded cabbage or coleslaw mix

2 medium fresh tomatoes, seeded and chopped

6 green onions, coarsely chopped

2 jalapeño peppers,* finely chopped

¼ cup apple cider vinegar

3 tablespoons honey

1 teaspoon salt

*Jalapeño peppers can sting and irritate the skin, so wear rubber gloves when handling peppers and do not touch your eyes.

Combine cabbage, tomatoes, green onions, jalapeño peppers, vinegar, honey and salt in serving bowl; mix well. Cover; chill at least 2 hours before serving.

TIP: For a milder coleslaw, discard the seeds and veins when chopping the jalapeño peppers. This is where much of the heat from the peppers is stored.

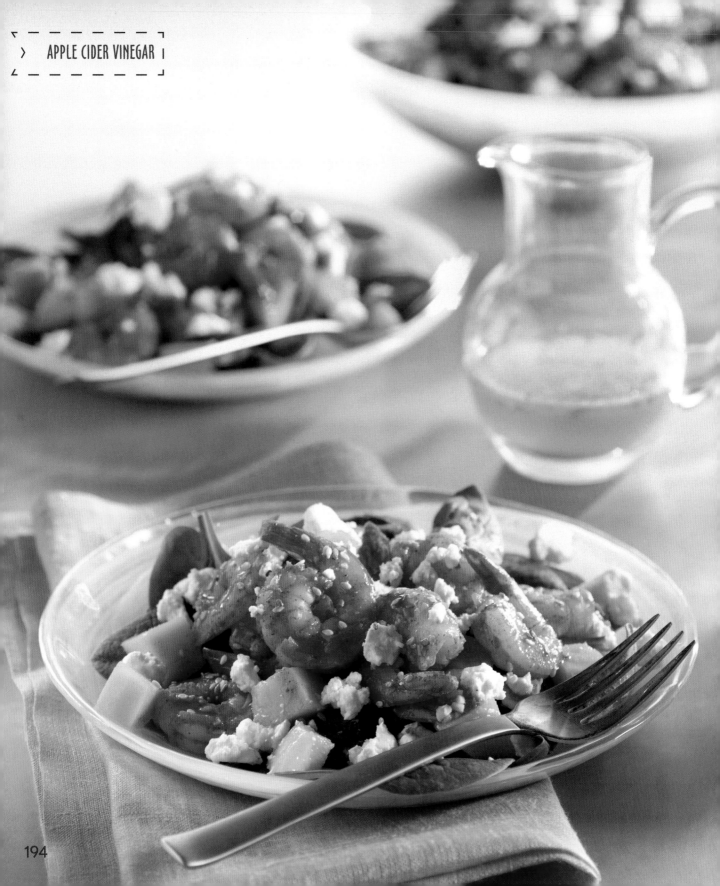

SPINACH SALAD WITH ORANGE-CHILI GLAZED SHRIMP
Makes 4 servings

Orange-Chili Glazed Shrimp (recipe follows)

¼ cup orange juice

1 tablespoon apple cider vinegar

2 teaspoons toasted sesame seeds*

1 clove garlic, minced

1 teaspoon grated orange peel

1 teaspoon olive oil

½ teaspoon honey

⅛ teaspoon red pepper flakes

12 cups packed fresh spinach

1 large ripe mango or medium ripe papaya, peeled and cored

½ cup (2 ounces) crumbled feta cheese

*To toast sesame seeds, spread in small skillet. Shake skillet over medium-low heat 2 minutes or until seeds begin to pop and turn golden brown.

1. Prepare Orange-Chili Glazed Shrimp. Set aside.

2. Combine orange juice, vinegar, sesame seeds, garlic, orange peel, oil, honey and red pepper flakes in small bowl; stir to blend. Set aside.

3. Place spinach leaves in large bowl; toss with dressing. Top with mango, cheese and Orange-Chili Glazed Shrimp.

ORANGE-CHILI GLAZED SHRIMP
Makes 4 servings

½ cup orange juice

4 cloves garlic, minced

1 teaspoon chili powder

8 ounces large raw shrimp, peeled, deveined

1. Combine orange juice, garlic and chili powder in large nonstick skillet. Bring to a boil over high heat. Boil 3 minutes or until mixture just coats bottom of skillet.

2. Reduce heat to medium. Add shrimp; cook and stir 2 minutes or until shrimp are pink and opaque. (Add additional orange juice or water to keep shrimp moist, if necessary.)

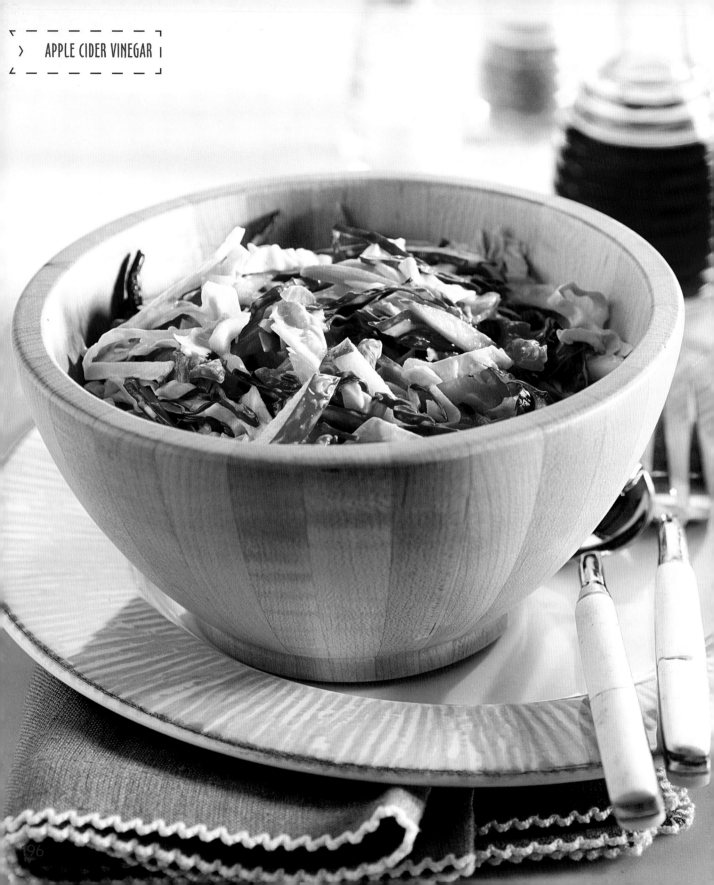

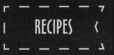

RED CABBAGE AND FRUIT SLAW
Makes 8 servings

- 2 cups shredded savoy cabbage
- ⅓ cup shredded carrot
- ⅓ cup dried apricots, cut into thin matchstick strips
- ⅓ cup thin apple strips
- ½ cup mayonnaise
- 3 tablespoons apple cider vinegar
- 1 to 3 tablespoons sugar
- 2 cups shredded red cabbage

1. Combine savoy cabbage, carrot, apricots and apple in large bowl; mix well.

2. Combine mayonnaise, vinegar and sugar in small bowl until well blended. Pour over cabbage mixture; toss to coat. Refrigerate at least 1 hour before serving. Just before serving, stir in red cabbage.

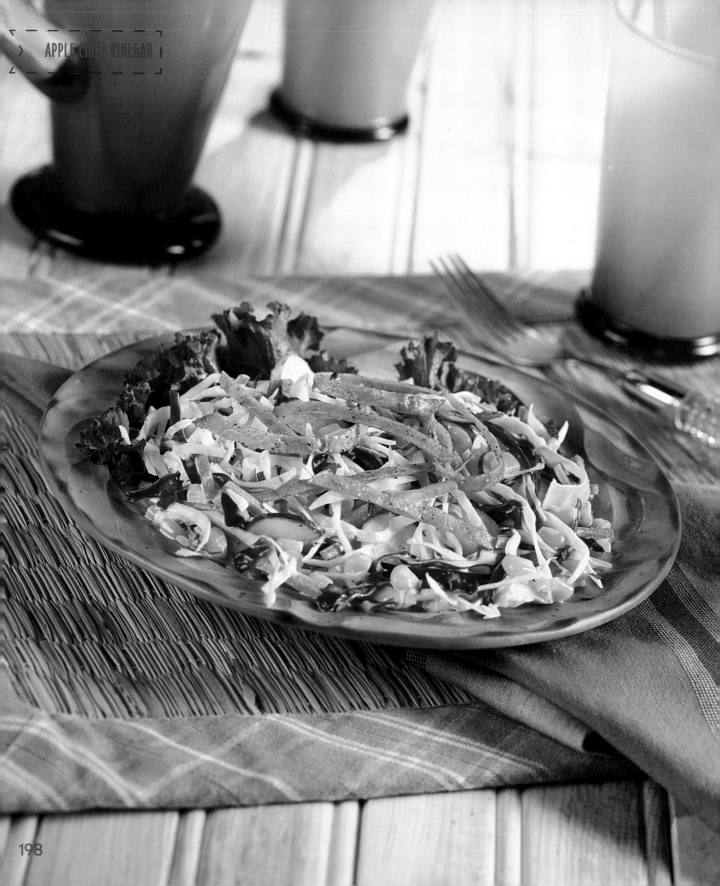

MEXICAN SLAW

Makes 8 servings

1   (6-inch) corn tortilla, cut into thin strips
     Nonstick cooking spray
¼   teaspoon chili powder
3   cups shredded green cabbage
1   cup shredded red cabbage
½   cup shredded carrots
½   cup sliced radishes
½   cup corn
¼   cup coarsely chopped fresh cilantro
¼   cup mayonnaise
1   tablespoon fresh lime juice
2   teaspoons apple cider vinegar
1   teaspoon honey
½   teaspoon ground cumin
     Salt and black pepper

1. Preheat oven to 350°F. Arrange tortilla strips in even layer on nonstick baking sheet. Spray strips with cooking spray and sprinkle with chili powder. Bake 6 to 8 minutes or until crisp.

2. Combine cabbage, carrots, radishes, corn and cilantro in large bowl. Combine mayonnaise, lime juice, vinegar, honey, cumin, salt and pepper in small bowl; stir to blend. Add mayonnaise mixture to cabbage mixture; toss gently to coat. Top with baked tortilla strips.

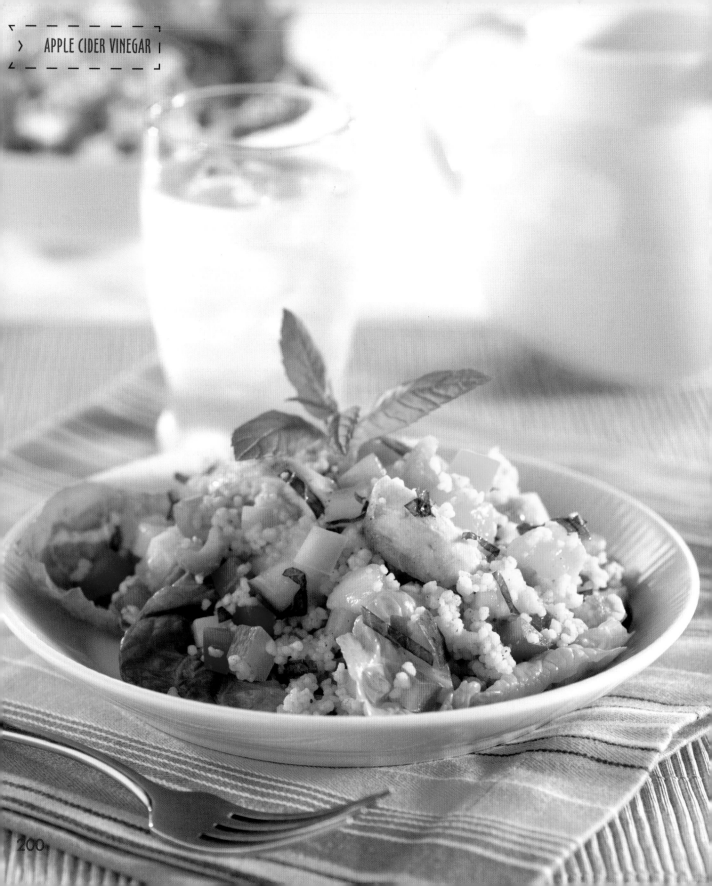

CHICKEN AND COUSCOUS SALAD

Makes 6 servings

1   can (about 14 ounces) chicken broth

½   teaspoon ground cinnamon

¼   teaspoon ground nutmeg

¼   teaspoon curry powder

1   cup uncooked couscous

1½   pounds boneless skinless chicken breasts, cooked and cut into ½-inch pieces

2   cups fresh pineapple chunks

2   cups diced seedless cucumber

2   cups diced red bell peppers

2   cups diced yellow bell peppers

1   cup sliced celery

½   cup sliced green onions

3   tablespoons water

3   tablespoons apple cider vinegar

2   tablespoons vegetable oil

1   tablespoon fresh mint leaves, plus additional for garnish

   Lettuce leaves (optional)

1. Combine broth, cinnamon, nutmeg and curry powder in large nonstick saucepan; bring to a boil over high heat. Stir in couscous; remove from heat. Let stand, covered, 5 minutes. Fluff couscous with fork; cool to room temperature.

2. Add chicken, pineapple, cucumber, bell peppers, celery and green onions to couscous; gently toss.

3. Whisk water, vinegar, oil and 1 tablespoon mint in small bowl until well blended. Pour over couscous mixture; gently toss to coat. Serve over lettuce, if desired. Garnish with additional mint.

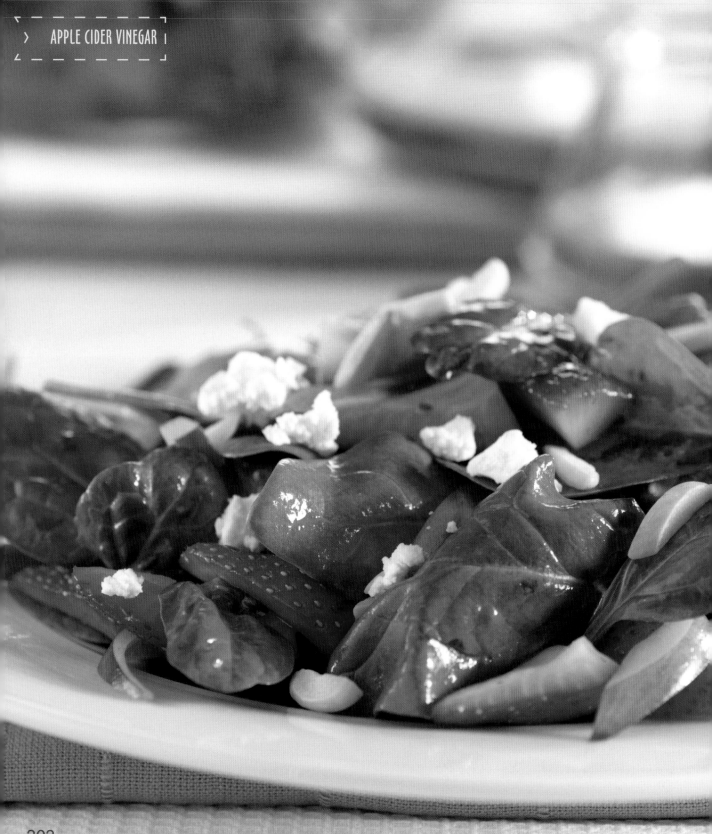

FRESH SPINACH-STRAWBERRY SALAD

Makes 5 servings

- 1 package (9 ounces) fresh spinach leaves
- ¾ cup thinly sliced red onion
- ⅓ cup pomegranate or pomegranate-cherry juice
- 3 tablespoons sugar
- 3 tablespoons apple cider vinegar
- 2 tablespoons vegetable oil
- 2 tablespoons toasted (dark) sesame oil
- 1 to 2 teaspoons grated fresh ginger (optional)
- ¼ teaspoon red pepper flakes
- ⅛ teaspoon salt
- 2 cups quartered hulled fresh strawberries
- 2 to 4 ounces slivered almonds, toasted*
- 4 ounces goat cheese, crumbled (optional)

*To toast almonds, cook and stir in small skillet over medium heat 1 to 2 minutes or until lightly browned.

1. Combine spinach and onion in large bowl. Combine pomegranate juice, sugar, vinegar, vegetable oil, sesame oil, ginger, if desired, red pepper flakes and salt in small jar; cover and shake vigorously until well blended.

2. Pour dressing over spinach and onion; toss to coat. Add strawberries; toss gently. Top with almonds and goat cheese, if desired. Serve immediately.

NOTE: The dressing may be prepared up to 2 days in advance and refrigerated. Shake well before using; toss with spinach just before serving.

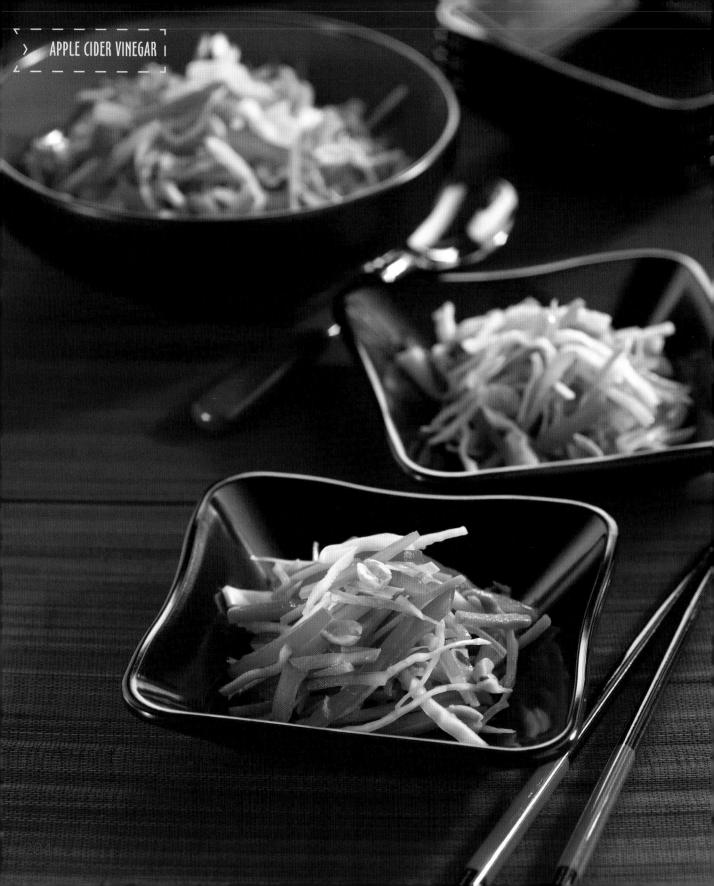

APPLE CIDER VINEGAR

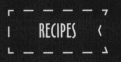

BRIGHT AND GINGERY CHINESE SLAW
Makes 6 servings

2   cups matchstick carrots

½   cup thinly shredded red cabbage

1   medium red bell pepper, cut into thin 2-inch strips

½   medium green bell pepper, cut into thin 2-inch strips

3   tablespoons soy sauce

3   tablespoons sugar

2   to 3 tablespoons apple cider vinegar

2   tablespoons dark sesame oil

1   tablespoon grated fresh ginger

¼   teaspoon red pepper flakes

½   cup peanuts, toasted*

*To toast peanuts, cook and stir in small skillet over medium heat 1 to 2 minutes or until lightly browned.

1. Combine carrots, cabbage and peppers in medium bowl; toss to blend.

2. Combine soy sauce, sugar, vinegar, oil, ginger and red pepper flakes in glass jar; seal lid. Shake vigorously to blend well. Pour dressing over car-rot mixture. Add peanuts; toss gently to coat.

VARIATION: If the sesame oil flavor is too strong, substitute 1 tablespoon canola oil for 1 tablespoon sesame oil.

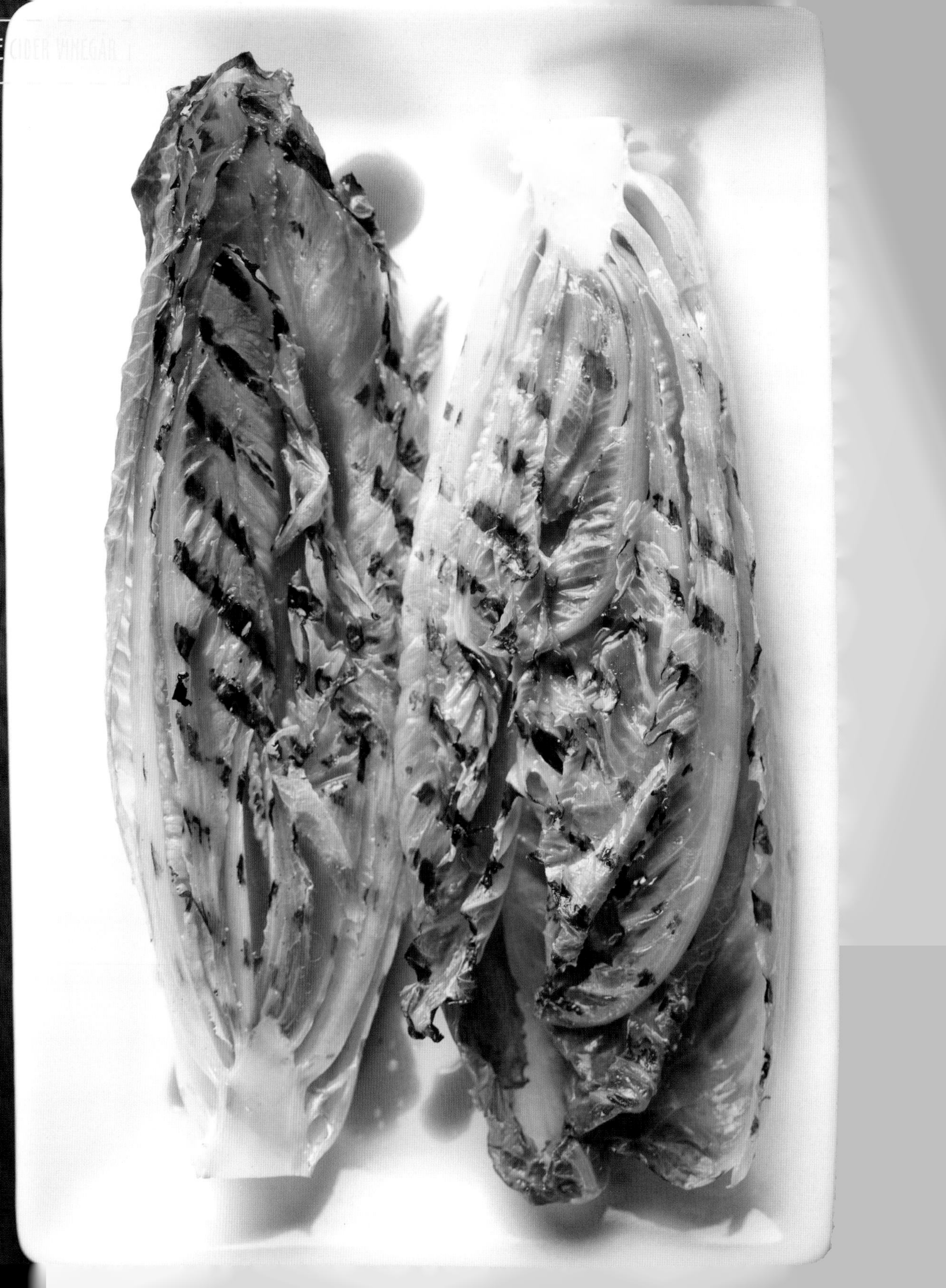

GRILLED ROMAINE HEARTS WITH TANGY VINAIGRETTE

Makes 6 servings, plus 1 quart vinaigrette

3	cups cola beverage
1/3	cup white vinegar
1/3	cup canola oil
1/4	cup sugar
1	teaspoon salt
1/2	teaspoon onion powder
1/2	teaspoon garlic powder
3	tablespoons ketchup
1	tablespoon balsamic vinegar
1/8	teaspoon black pepper
2	tablespoons honey mustard
6	romaine hearts
1/4	to 1/2 cup olive oil
	Salt and black pepper

1. Combine cola, white vinegar, canola oil, sugar, 1 teaspoon salt, onion powder, garlic powder, ketchup, balsamic vinegar, 1/8 teaspoon pepper and mustard in medium bowl; stir to blend. Set aside.

2. Prepare grill for direct cooking over medium-high heat. Cut romaine hearts in half lengthwise; drizzle with olive oil and sprinkle generously with salt and pepper.

3. Grill about 2 minutes per side or until wilted and lightly charred.

4. Drizzle with vinaigrette. Refrigerate remaining vinaigrette for another use.

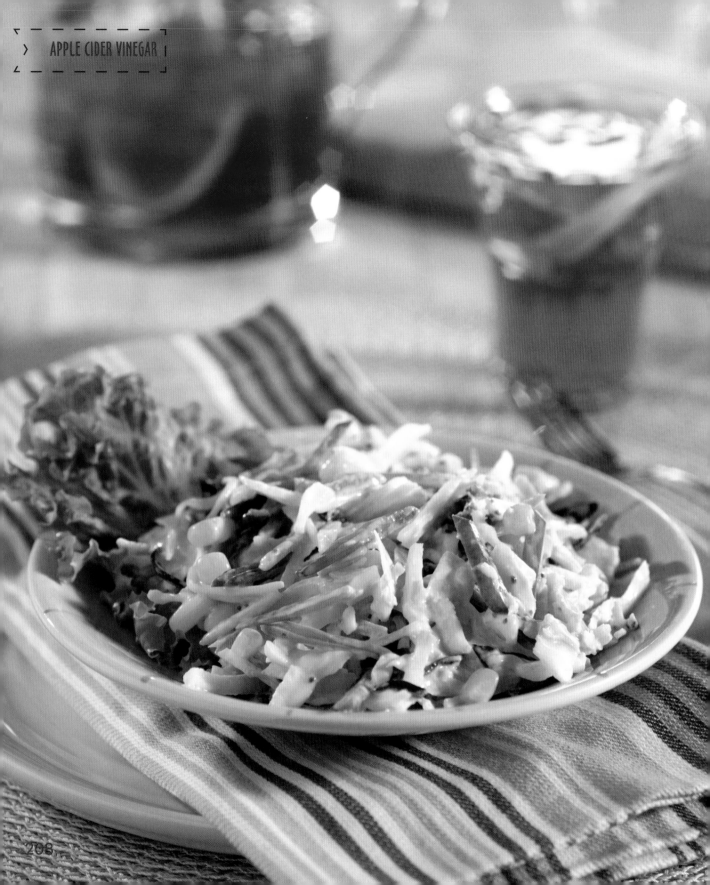

COLESLAW WITH SNOW PEAS AND CORN
Makes 4 servings

4 cups (about 8 ounces) coleslaw mix

½ cup trimmed vertically sliced snow peas

½ cup whole kernel corn

¼ cup mayonnaise

¼ cup sour cream

¼ cup buttermilk

1 tablespoon apple cider vinegar

2 teaspoons sugar

¼ teaspoon celery seed

1. Combine coleslaw, snow peas and corn in large bowl; toss to blend.

2. Whisk mayonnaise, sour cream, buttermilk, vinegar, sugar and celery seed in medium bowl. Add to coleslaw mixture; toss to blend.

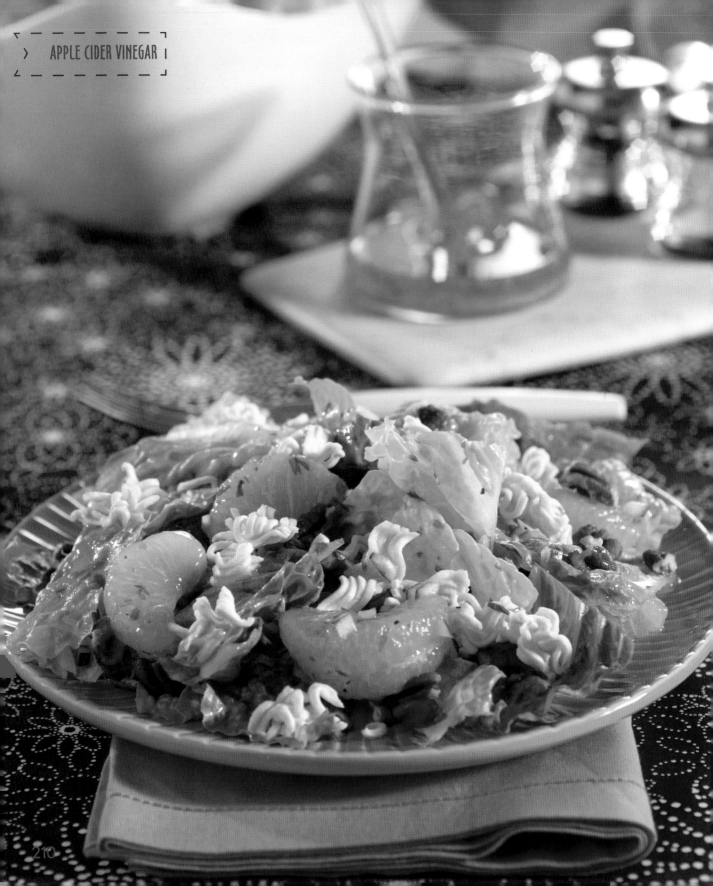

MANDARIN SALAD

Makes 4 servings

⅓ cup olive oil

2 tablespoons apple cider vinegar

2 teaspoons honey

2 teaspoons dried tarragon

½ teaspoon dry mustard

Salt and black pepper

1 can (11 ounces) mandarin oranges, drained, and 1 tablespoon juice reserved

4 cups chopped romaine lettuce

1 package (3 ounces) ramen noodles, any flavor, lightly crumbled*

½ cup toasted pecans, coarsely chopped**

¼ cup chopped red onion

*Discard seasoning packet.

**To toast pecans, spread in single layer in small heavy skillet. Cook and stir over medium heat 1 to 2 minutes or until nuts are lightly browned. Remove from skillet immediately. Cool before using.

1. Whisk oil, vinegar, honey, tarragon, mustard, salt, pepper and reserved mandarin orange juice in large bowl.

2. Add lettuce, oranges, crumbled noodles, pecans and onion to dressing; toss to combine.

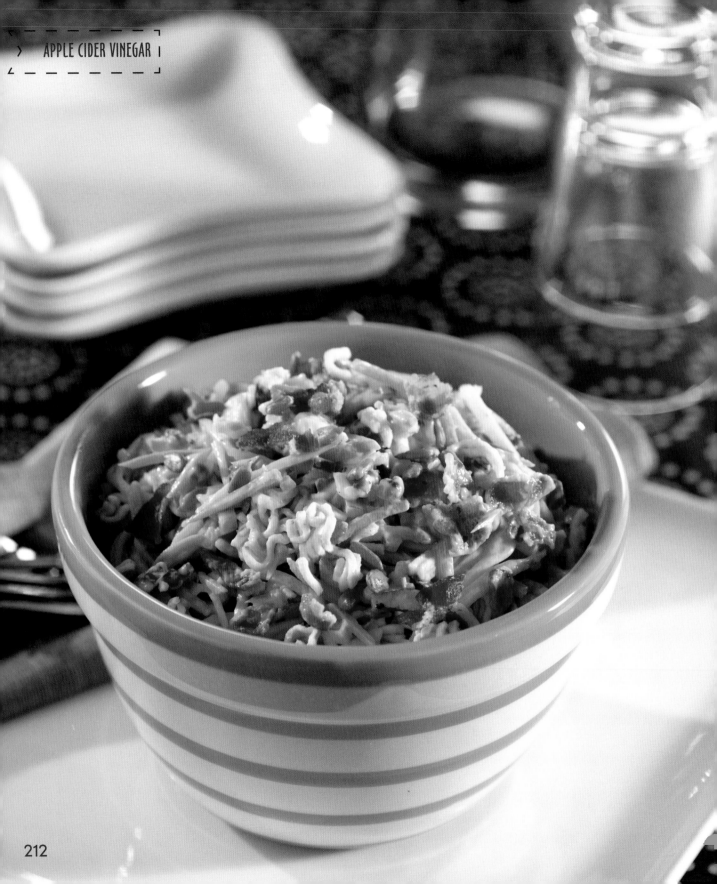

BROCCOLI SLAW

Makes 6 to 8 servings

- 1 package (12 ounces) broccoli slaw
- 6 slices bacon, crisp-cooked and crumbled
- ½ small red onion, chopped
- 1 package (3 ounces) ramen noodles, any flavor, crumbled and divided*
- ¼ cup roasted salted sunflower seeds
- 1 cup mayonnaise
- 2 tablespoons sugar
- 2 tablespoons apple cider vinegar
- ¼ teaspoon black pepper

*Discard seasoning packet.

1. Combine broccoli slaw, bacon, onion, half of noodles and sunflower seeds in large bowl.

2. Whisk mayonnaise, sugar, vinegar and pepper in small bowl. Pour over slaw mixture; stir to combine. Garnish with remaining noodles. Serve immediately.

VARIATIONS: Any chopped nuts, such as peanuts or almonds, can be substituted for the sunflower seeds.

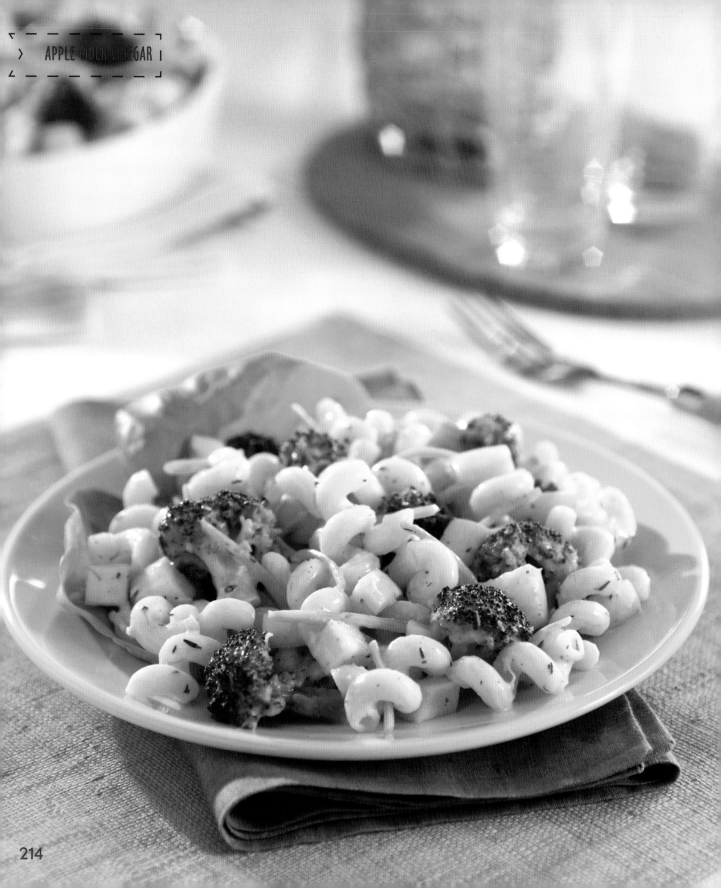

SWEET AND SOUR BROCCOLI PASTA SALAD

Makes 6 servings

8 ounces uncooked pasta twists

2 cups broccoli florets

⅓ cup shredded carrots

1 medium Red or Golden Delicious apple, cored, seeded and chopped

⅓ cup plain nonfat yogurt

⅓ cup apple juice

3 tablespoons apple cider vinegar

1 tablespoon olive oil

1 tablespoon Dijon mustard

1 teaspoon honey

½ teaspoon dried thyme

Lettuce leaves

1. Cook pasta according to package directions, omitting salt; add broccoli during last 2 minutes of cooking. Drain; rinse under cold running water until pasta and broccoli are cool.

2. Combine pasta, broccoli, carrots and apple in medium bowl. Whisk yogurt, apple juice, vinegar, oil, mustard, honey and thyme in small bowl until smooth and well blended. Pour over pasta mixture; toss to coat.

3. Line six plates with lettuce. Top evenly with pasta salad.

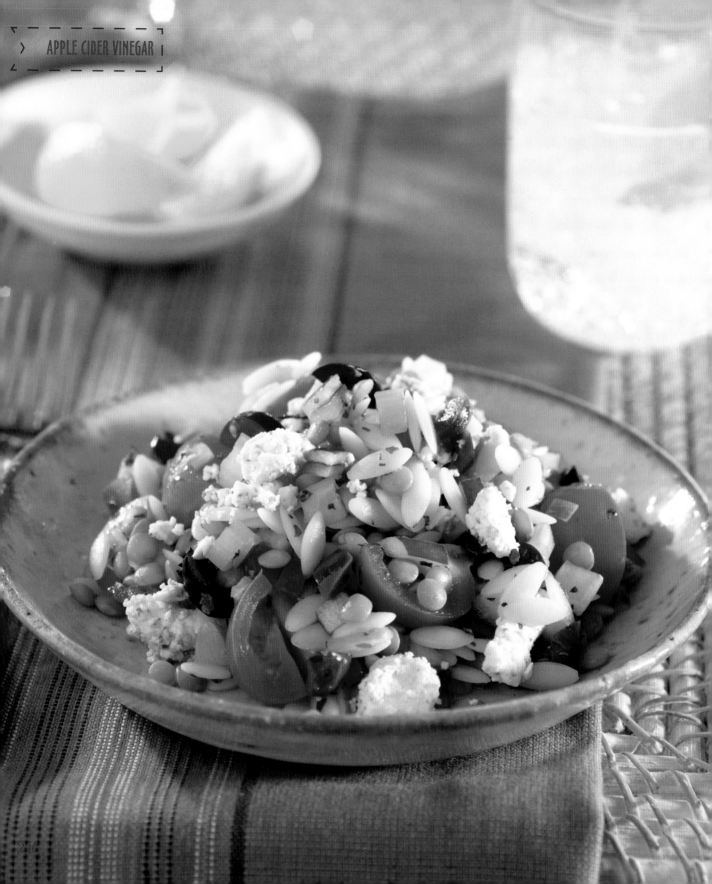

LENTIL AND ORZO PASTA SALAD

Makes 4 servings

8 cups water

½ cup dried lentils, rinsed and sorted

4 ounces uncooked orzo

1½ cups quartered cherry tomatoes, sweet grape variety

¾ cup finely chopped celery

½ cup chopped red onion

2 ounces pitted olives (about 16 olives), coarsely chopped

3 to 4 tablespoons apple cider vinegar

1 tablespoon olive oil

1 tablespoon dried basil

1 medium clove garlic, minced

⅛ teaspoon dried red pepper flakes

4 ounces feta cheese with sun-dried tomatoes and basil

1. Bring water to boil in Dutch oven over high heat. Add lentils; boil 12 minutes.

2. Add orzo; cook 10 minutes or just until tender. Drain. Rinse under cold water to cool completely. Drain well.

3. Meanwhile, combine tomatoes, celery, onion, olives, vinegar, oil, basil, garlic and red pepper flakes in large bowl; set aside.

4. Add lentil mixture to tomato mixture; toss gently to blend. Add cheese; toss gently. Let stand 15 minutes before serving.

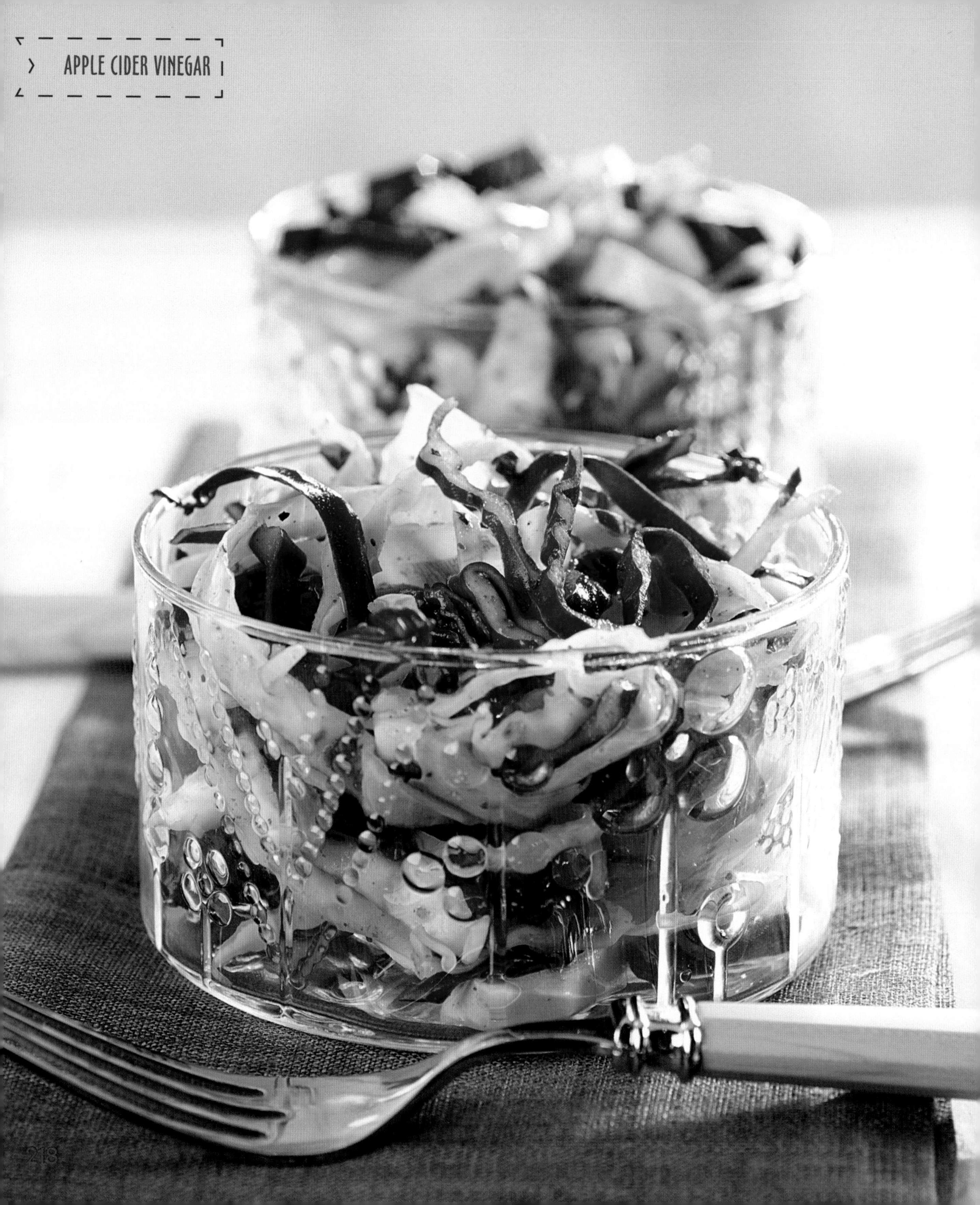

LEMONY CABBAGE SLAW WITH CURRY
Makes 6 servings

~~~~~~~~~~~~~~~~~~~~~~~~~~~~

4   cups shredded green or white cabbage

2   tablespoons chopped green bell pepper

2   tablespoons chopped red bell pepper

1   green onion, thinly sliced

2   tablespoons apple cider vinegar

1   tablespoon lemon juice

1   tablespoon sugar

1   teaspoon curry powder

½   teaspoon salt

½   teaspoon celery seeds

    Green and red bell pepper rings (optional)

1. Combine cabbage, chopped bell peppers and green onion in large bowl. Combine vinegar, lemon juice, sugar, curry powder, salt and celery seeds in small bowl; stir to blend. Pour vinegar mixture over cabbage mixture; mix well.

2. Refrigerate, covered, at least 4 hours or overnight, stirring occasionally. Garnish with bell pepper rings.

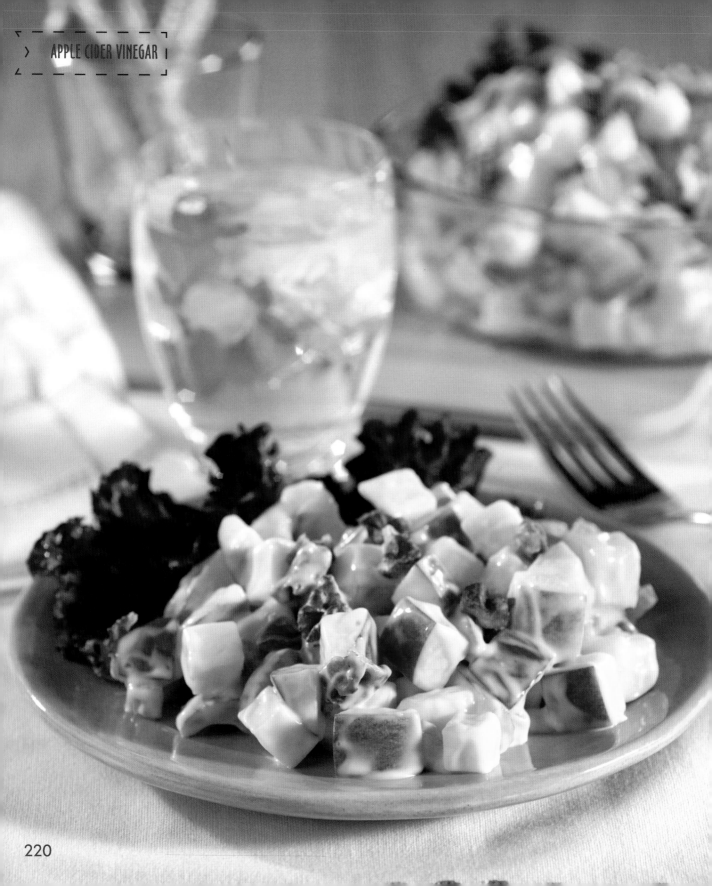

CHEESY WALDORF SALAD

Makes 6 to 8 servings

⅓ cup mayonnaise

1 tablespoon honey

1 tablespoon apple cider vinegar

4 small *or* 3 large apples, cored and cut into ½-inch pieces (about 4 cups)

4 ounces provolone cheese, cubed

2 stalks celery, thinly sliced

½ cup walnuts or pecans, toasted* and chopped, divided

Red leaf lettuce leaves

1. Combine mayonnaise, honey and vinegar in large bowl; stir to blend. Add apples, cheese, celery and ¼ cup walnuts; stir to coat. (At this point the salad may be refrigerated up to 8 hours.)

2. To serve, line individual plates with lettuce; top with salad. Sprinkle remaining ¼ cup walnuts over each serving.

*To toast walnuts, spread in single layer in small heavy skillet. Cook and stir over medium heat 1 to 2 minutes or until nuts are lightly browned. Remove from skillet immediately. Cool before using.

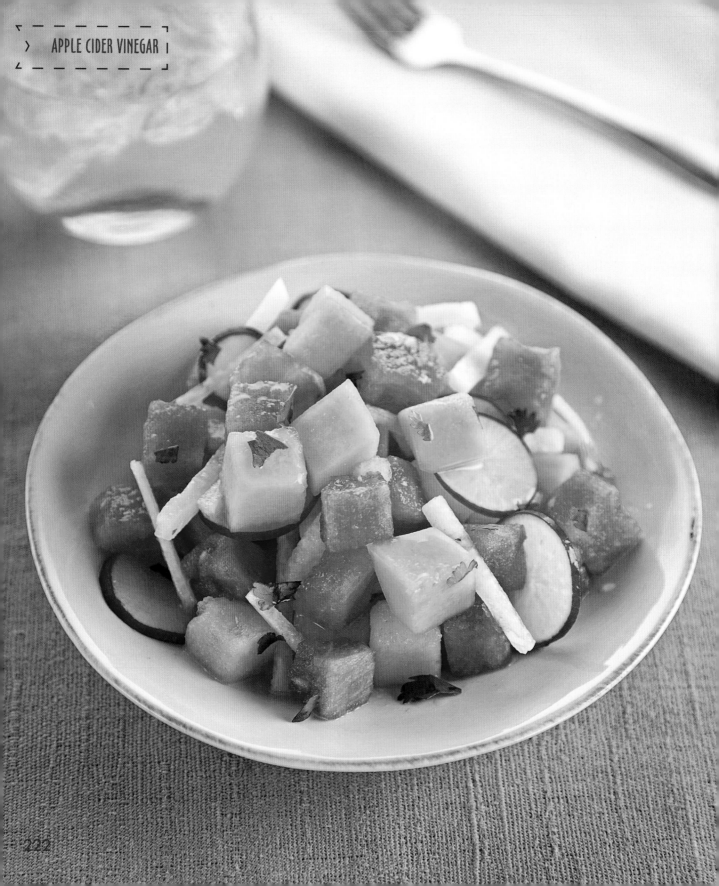

CRUNCHY JICAMA, RADISH AND MELON SALAD
Makes 8 servings

- 3 cups thinly cut jicama
- 3 cups watermelon cubes
- 2 cups cantaloupe cubes
- 1 cup sliced radishes
- 3 tablespoons chopped fresh cilantro
- 2 tablespoons olive oil
- 2 tablespoons lime juice
- 1 tablespoon orange juice
- 1 tablespoon apple cider vinegar
- 1 tablespoon honey
- ½ teaspoon salt

1. Combine jicama, watermelon, cantaloupe and radishes in large bowl; gently mix.

2. Whisk cilantro, oil, lime juice, orange juice, vinegar, honey and salt in small bowl until smooth and well blended. Add to salad; gently toss to coat. Serve immediately.

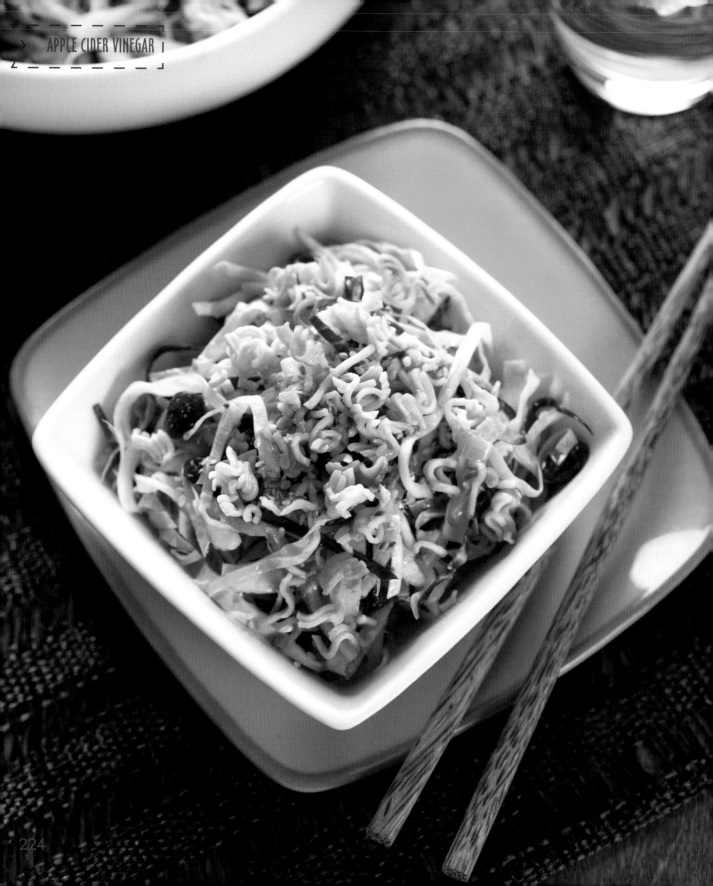

ORANGE-GINGER RAMEN SLAW

Makes 6 to 8 servings

1   package (3 ounces) ramen noodles, any flavor, coarsely crumbled*

1   tablespoon sesame seeds

6   cups finely shredded green cabbage

2   cups shredded carrots

½   cup diced red onion

½   cup raisins

¾   cup orange marmalade, microwaved for 30 seconds

¼   cup apple cider vinegar

¼   cup canola oil

3   tablespoons grated fresh ginger

1   tablespoon soy sauce

1   teaspoon grated orange peel (optional)

1   teaspoon hot pepper sauce *or* ¼ teaspoon red pepper flakes (optional)

¼   teaspoon salt

*Discard seasoning packet.

1. Heat medium skillet over medium-high heat. Add ramen noodles and sesame seeds; cook and stir 2 minutes or until lightly browned. Set aside on large plate.

2. Combine cabbage, carrots, onion, raisins, marmalade, vinegar, oil, ginger, soy sauce, orange peel, hot pepper sauce, if desired, and salt in large bowl; toss to blend. Cover; refrigerate 20 minutes.

3. Sprinkle with toasted ramen and sesame seed mixture just before serving.

VARIATION: Add leftover diced cooked chicken for a main-dish salad.

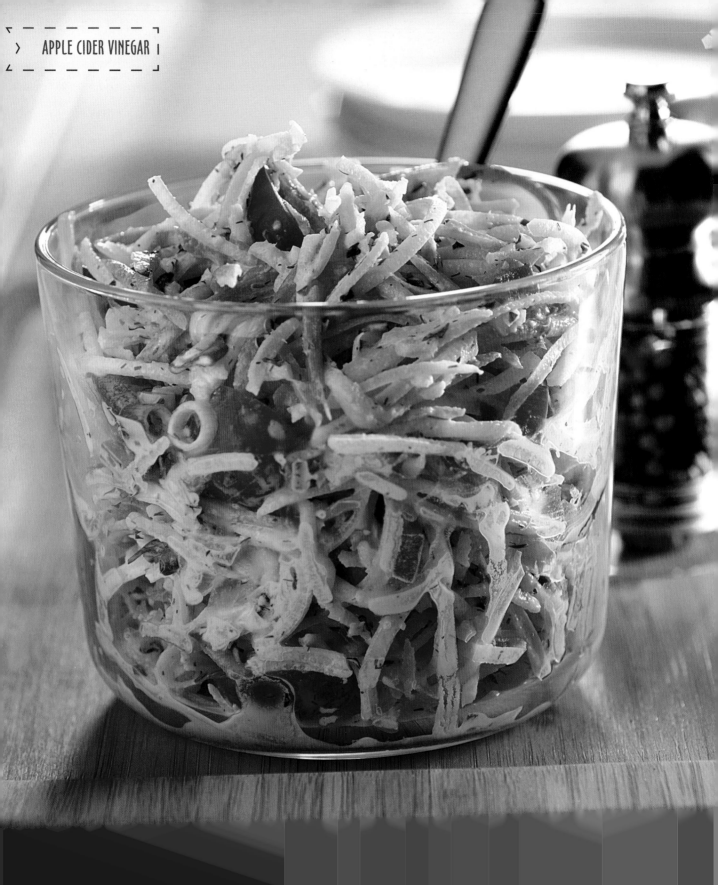

KOHLRABI AND CARROT SLAW
Makes 8 servings

2   pounds kohlrabi bulbs, peeled

2   medium carrots, shredded

1   small red bell pepper, chopped

8   cherry tomatoes, halved

2   green onions, thinly sliced

¼   cup mayonnaise

¼   cup plain yogurt

2   tablespoons apple cider vinegar

2   tablespoons finely chopped fresh parsley

1   teaspoon dried dill weed

¼   teaspoon salt

¼   teaspoon ground cumin

⅛   teaspoon black pepper

1. Spiral kohlrabi with thick spiral blade; cut into desired lengths.

2. Combine kohlrabi, carrots, bell pepper, tomatoes and green onions in medium bowl.

3. Combine mayonnaise, yogurt, vinegar, parsley, dill weed, salt, cumin and black pepper in small bowl; stir until smooth. Add to vegetables; toss to coat. Cover; refrigerate until ready to serve.

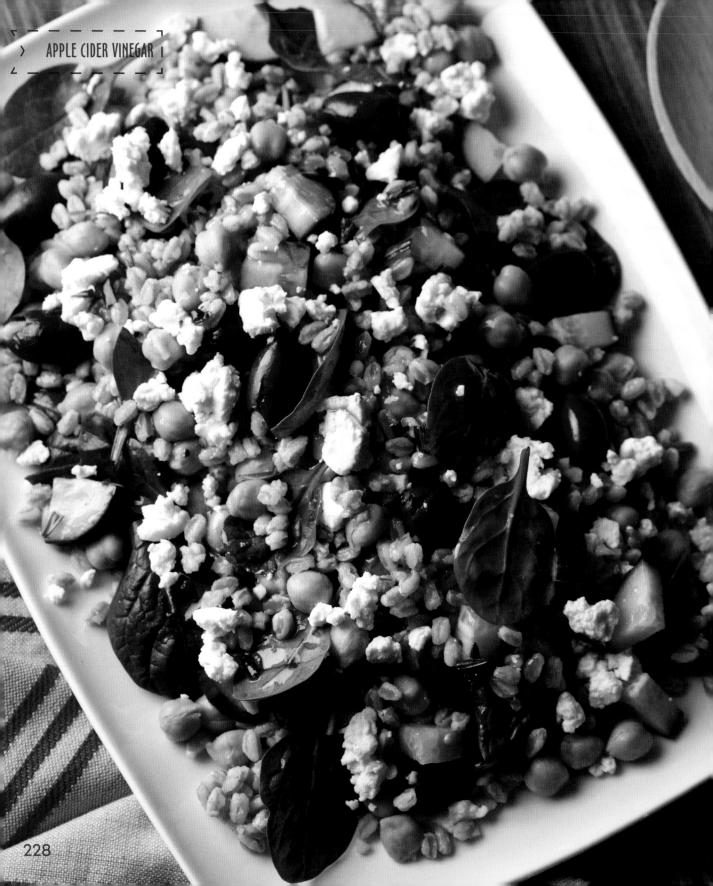

FARRO, CHICKPEA AND SPINACH SALAD

Makes 4 to 6 salads

- 1 cup uncooked pearled farro
- 3 cups baby spinach, stemmed
- 1 medium cucumber, chopped
- 1 can (15 ounces) chickpeas, rinsed and drained
- ¾ cup pitted kalamata olives
- ¼ cup extra virgin olive oil
- 3 tablespoons apple cider vinegar mixed with ½ teaspoon sugar
- 1 teaspoon chopped fresh rosemary
- 1 clove garlic, minced
- 1 teaspoon salt
- ⅛ to ¼ teaspoon red pepper flakes (optional)
- ½ cup crumbled goat or feta cheese

1. Bring 4 cups water to a boil in medium saucepan. Add farro; reduce heat and simmer 20 to 25 minutes or until farro is tender. Drain and rinse under cold water until cool.

2. Meanwhile, combine spinach, cucumber, chickpeas, olives, oil, vinegar, rosemary, garlic, salt and red pepper flakes, if desired, in large bowl. Stir in farro until well blended. Add cheese; toss gently.

ON THE SIDE

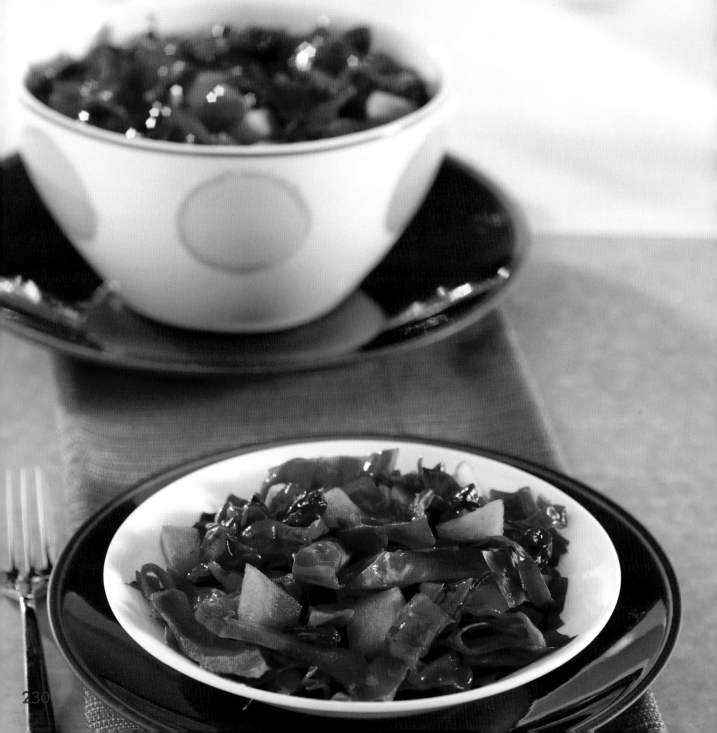

BRAISED SWEET AND SOUR CABBAGE AND APPLES
Makes 4 to 6 servings

- 2 tablespoons unsalted butter
- 6 cups coarsely shredded red cabbage
- 1 large sweet apple, peeled and cut into 1-inch pieces
- ½ cup raisins
- ½ cup apple cider
- 3 tablespoons apple cider vinegar, divided
- 2 tablespoons packed dark brown sugar
  Salt and black pepper
- 3 whole cloves

SLOW COOKER DIRECTIONS
1. Melt butter in large skillet over medium heat. Add cabbage; cook and stir 3 minutes until glossy. Remove to slow cooker.

2. Add apple, raisins, apple cider, 2 tablespoons vinegar, brown sugar, salt, pepper and cloves. Cover; cook on LOW 2½ to 3 hours.

3. To serve, remove and discard cloves. Stir in remaining 1 tablespoon vinegar.

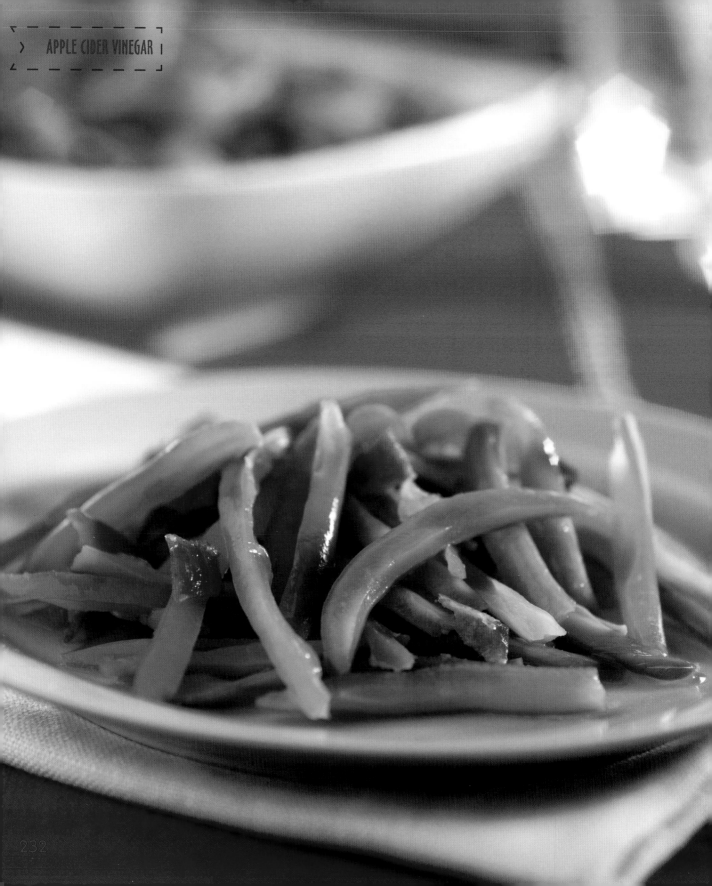

GREEN BEANS WITH MAPLE-BACON DRESSING
Makes 6 servings

- ½ cup chicken broth
- 1 bag (16 ounces) frozen French-style green beans
- 1 tablespoon bacon bits
- 1 tablespoon maple syrup
- 1 tablespoon apple cider vinegar
- ¼ teaspoon black pepper

1. Bring broth to a boil in large saucepan. Add beans; cover and simmer over medium heat about 7 minutes or until beans are crisp-tender. Drain; place beans in large bowl.

2. Combine bacon bits, maple syrup, vinegar and pepper in small bowl; stir to blend. Pour over beans; toss to coat.

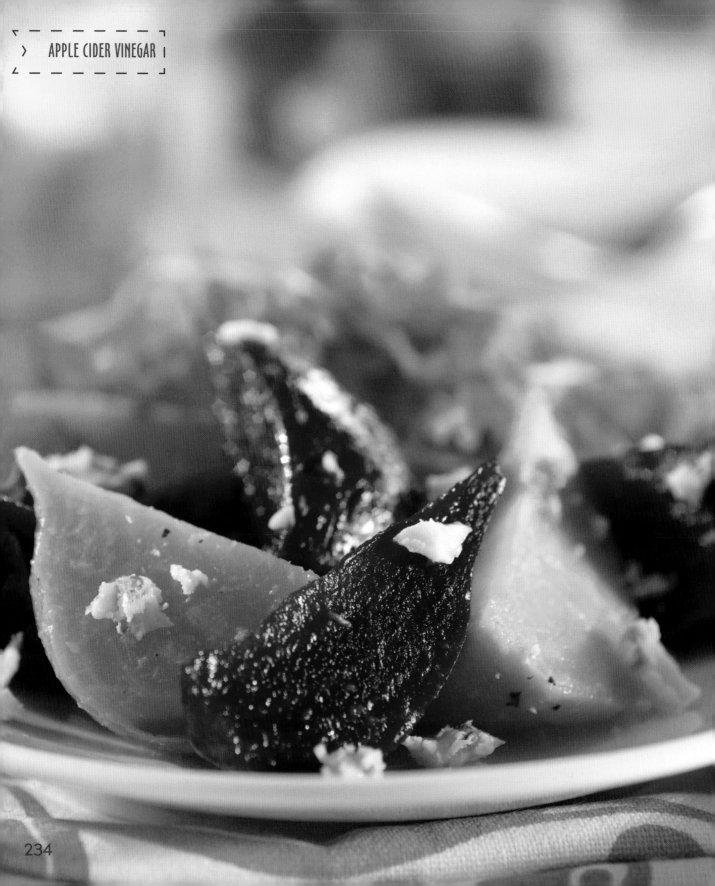

CIDER VINAIGRETTE-GLAZED BEETS
Makes 8 servings

6　medium beets

1　tablespoon olive oil

1　tablespoon apple cider vinegar

½　teaspoon prepared horseradish

½　teaspoon Dijon mustard

¼　teaspoon packed brown sugar

⅓　cup crumbled blue cheese (optional)

1. Cut tops off beets, leaving at least 1 inch of stems. Scrub beets under running water with soft vegetable brush, being careful not to break skins. Place beets in large saucepan; add water to cover. Bring to a boil over high heat. Reduce heat to low; simmer 30 minutes or just until beets are barely firm when pierced with fork. Remove to plate to cool slightly.

2. Meanwhile, whisk oil, vinegar, horseradish, mustard and brown sugar in medium bowl until well blended.

3. When beets are cool enough to handle, peel off skins and trim off root end. Cut beets into halves, then into wedges. Add warm beets to vinaigrette; gently toss to coat. Sprinkle with cheese, if desired. Serve warm or at room temperature.

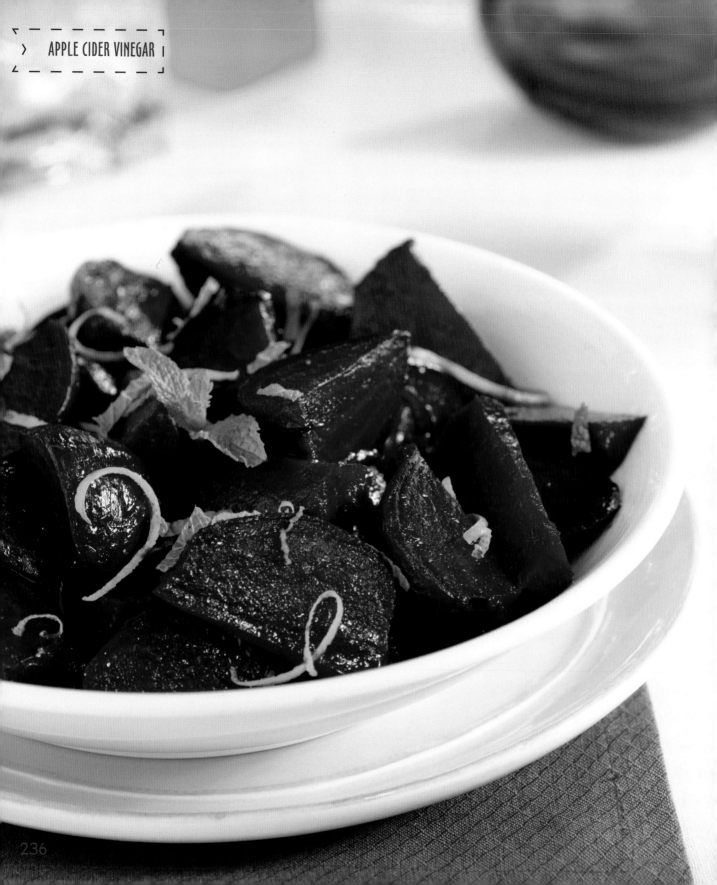

ORANGE AND MAPLE GLAZED ROASTED BEETS

Makes 4 servings

4 medium beets, scrubbed

2 teaspoons olive oil

¼ cup orange juice

3 tablespoons apple cider vinegar

2 tablespoons maple syrup

2 teaspoons grated orange peel, divided

1 teaspoon Dijon mustard

1 to 2 tablespoons chopped fresh mint (optional)

Salt and black pepper

1. Preheat oven to 425°F.

2. Place beets in glass baking dish. Drizzle with oil; toss to coat evenly. Cover; bake 45 minutes to 1 hour or until knife inserted into largest beet goes in easily. Let stand until cool enough to handle.

3. Peel and cut beets in half lengthwise; cut into wedges. Return to baking dish.

4. Whisk orange juice, vinegar, syrup, 1 teaspoon orange peel and mustard in small bowl until well blended. Pour over beets.

5. Bake 10 to 15 minutes or until heated through and all liquid is absorbed. Sprinkle with remaining 1 teaspoon orange peel and mint, if desired. Season with salt and pepper.

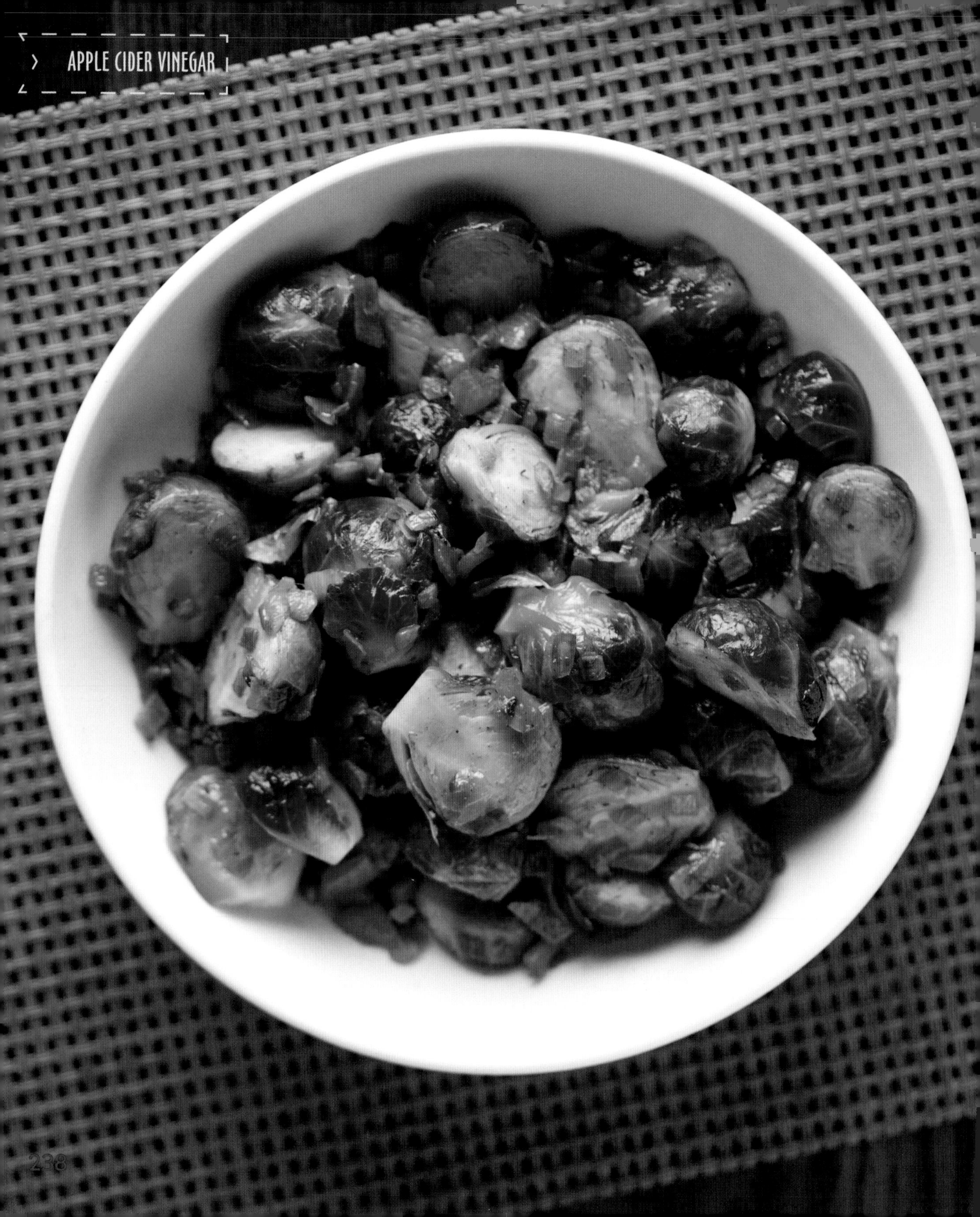

BRAISED BRUSSELS SPROUTS WITH CARAMELIZED ONIONS

Makes 4 servings

1 pound Brussels sprouts, trimmed and halved lengthwise

1½ teaspoons butter

1 cup diced onion

5 tablespoons cola beverage, divided

1 teaspoon balsamic vinegar

3 tablespoons dry white wine, divided

Salt and black pepper

1. Fill medium saucepan with Brussels sprouts and enough water to cover. Bring to a boil over high heat. Cook 5 minutes; drain.

2. Heat butter in large skillet over medium heat. Reduce heat to medium-low. Add onion; cook 10 minutes. Add 1 tablespoon cola and vinegar; cook 5 minutes.

3. Add Brussels sprouts to skillet with onions. Increase heat to medium. Add 2 tablespoons wine and 2 tablespoons cola; cook 3 minutes or until most liquid has evaporated from skillet.

4. Add remaining 1 tablespoon wine and 2 tablespoons cola to skillet; cook and stir 2 minutes or until most liquid has evaporated from pan and Brussels sprouts are tender. Season with salt and pepper.

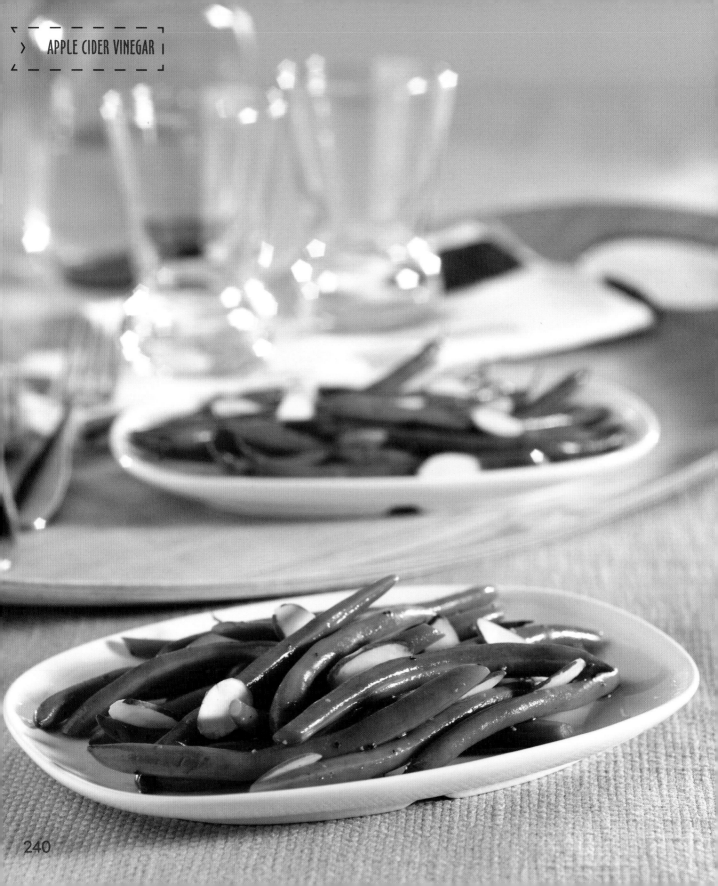

BALSAMIC GREEN BEANS WITH ALMONDS
Makes 4 servings

- 1   pound fresh green beans, trimmed
- 2   teaspoons olive oil
- 2   teaspoons balsamic vinegar
- ½   teaspoon salt
- ¼   teaspoon black pepper
- 2   tablespoons sliced almonds, toasted*

1. Place beans in medium saucepan; cover with water. Bring to a simmer over high heat. Reduce heat; simmer, uncovered, 4 to 8 minutes or until beans are crisp-tender. Drain well and return to saucepan.

2. Add oil, vinegar, salt and pepper; toss to coat. Sprinkle with almonds.

*To toast almonds, cook and stir in small skillet over medium heat 1 to 2 minutes or until lightly browned.

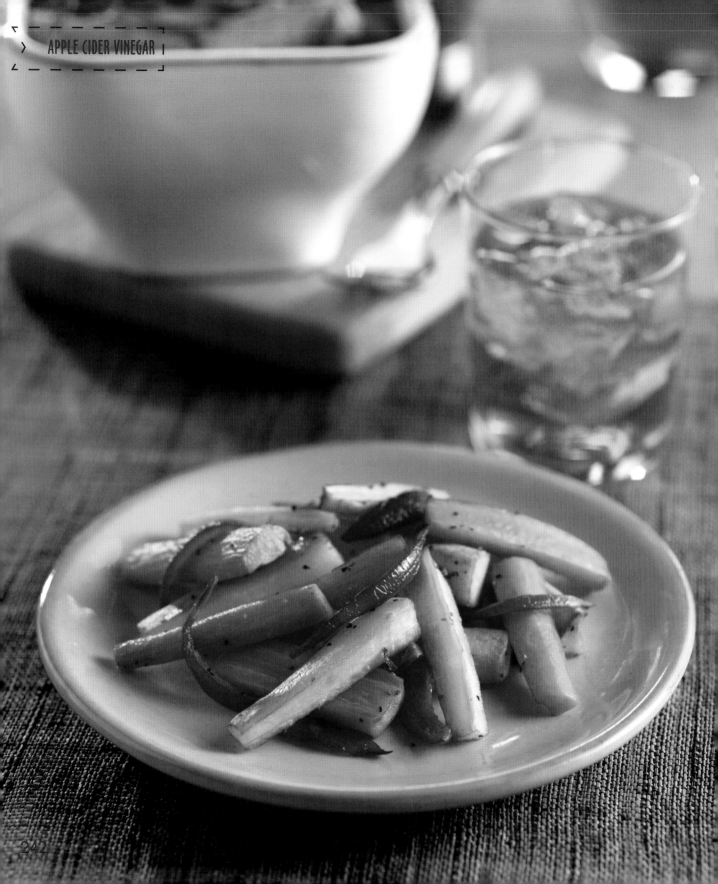

ROASTED PARSNIPS, CARROTS AND RED ONION
Makes 4 servings

2   carrots (9 ounces), cut into 2-inch-long pieces

2   parsnips (9 ounces), cut into 2-inch-long pieces

¾   cup vertically sliced red onion (¼-inch slices)

1   tablespoon balsamic vinegar

2   teaspoons extra virgin olive oil

¼   teaspoon salt

⅛   teaspoon black pepper

1. Preheat oven to 425°F. Line large baking sheet with foil or spray with nonstick cooking spray.

2. Combine carrots, parsnips, onion, vinegar, oil, salt and pepper in large bowl; toss to coat. Spread in single layer on prepared baking sheet.

3. Roast 25 minutes or until vegetables are tender, stirring occasionally.

NOTE: Parsnips are a pale white root vegetable similar to the carrot in shape. The parsnip, however, is broader at the top and has a smoother skin. The longer it stays in the ground, the sweeter it becomes. Choose parsnips that are firm, unblemished, and small or medium in size (about 8 inches long). Rinse and scrub parsnips with a vegetable brush to remove embedded soil. Peel parsnips with a swivel-bladed vegetable peeler or paring knife. Trim off ends and discard. For even cooking, parsnips are best chopped, cubed, sliced, or cut into strips before cooking.

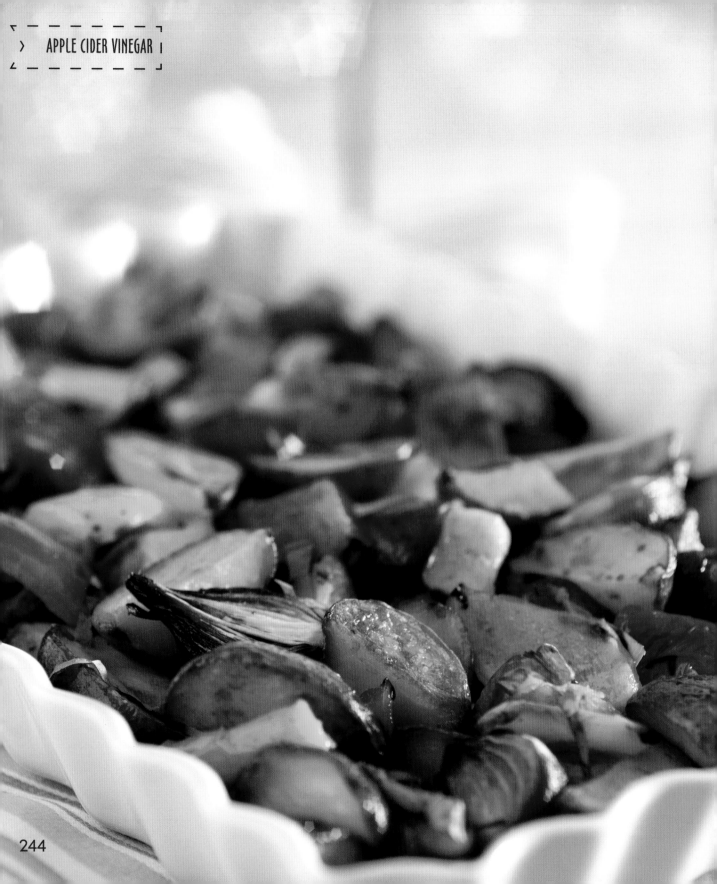

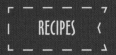

MEDITERRANEAN-STYLE ROASTED VEGETABLES
Makes 6 servings

1½ pounds red potatoes, cut into ½-inch pieces

1 tablespoon plus 1½ teaspoons olive oil, divided

1 red bell pepper, cut into ½-inch pieces

1 yellow or orange bell pepper, cut into ½-inch pieces

1 small red onion, cut into ½-inch wedges

2 cloves garlic, minced

½ teaspoon salt

¼ teaspoon black pepper

1 tablespoon balsamic vinegar

¼ cup chopped fresh basil leaves

1. Preheat oven to 425°F. Spray large roasting pan with nonstick cooking spray.

2. Place potatoes in prepared pan. Drizzle with 1 tablespoon oil; toss to coat evenly. Roast 10 minutes.

3. Add bell peppers and onion to pan. Drizzle with remaining 1½ teaspoons oil. Sprinkle with garlic, salt and black pepper; toss to coat evenly. Roast 18 to 20 minutes or until vegetables are browned and tender, stirring once.

4. Remove vegetables to large serving dish. Drizzle vinegar over vegetables; toss to coat. Add basil; toss to blend. Serve warm or at room temperature.

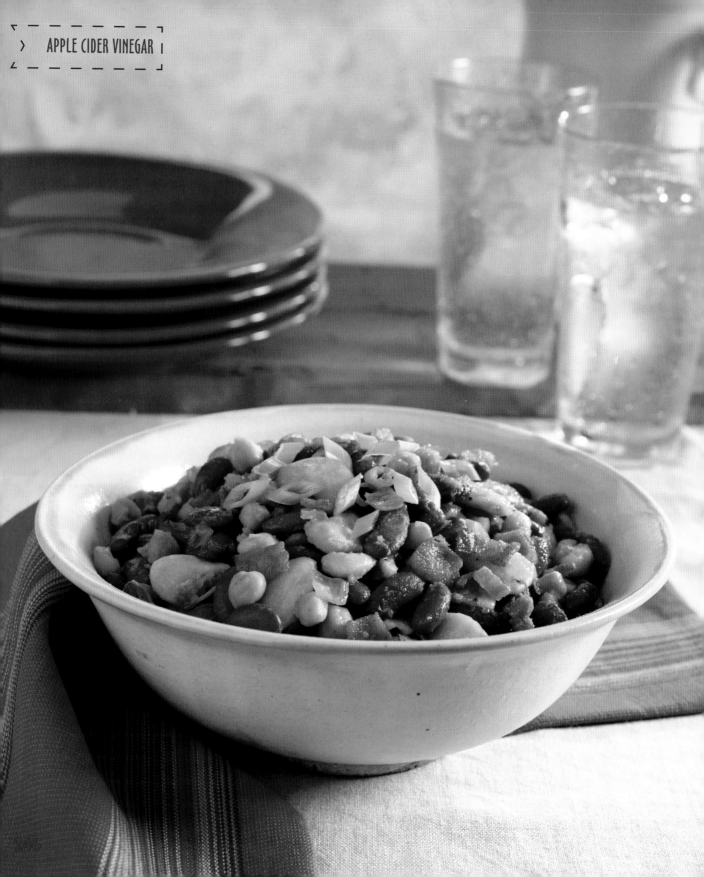

FIVE-BEAN CASSEROLE
Makes 16 servings

- 2 onions, chopped
- 8 ounces bacon, diced
- 2 cloves garlic, minced
- ½ cup packed brown sugar
- ½ cup apple cider vinegar
- 1 teaspoon salt
- 1 teaspoon ground mustard
- ¼ teaspoon black pepper
- 2 cans (about 15 ounces each) kidney beans, rinsed and drained
- 1 can (about 15 ounces) chickpeas, rinsed and drained
- 1 can (about 15 ounces) butter beans, rinsed and drained
- 1 can (about 15 ounces) Great Northern or cannellini beans, rinsed and drained
- 1 can (about 15 ounces) baked beans

   Chopped green onions (optional)

SLOW COOKER DIRECTIONS

1. Combine onions, bacon and garlic in large skillet over medium heat; cook and stir 6 to 8 minutes or until onions are tender. Drain. Stir in brown sugar, vinegar, salt, mustard and pepper. Reduce heat to low; simmer 15 minutes.

2. Combine beans in slow cooker; stir to blend. Spoon onion mixture evenly over top. Cover; cook on LOW 6 to 8 hours or on HIGH 3 to 4 hours. Sprinkle with green onions just before serving, if desired.

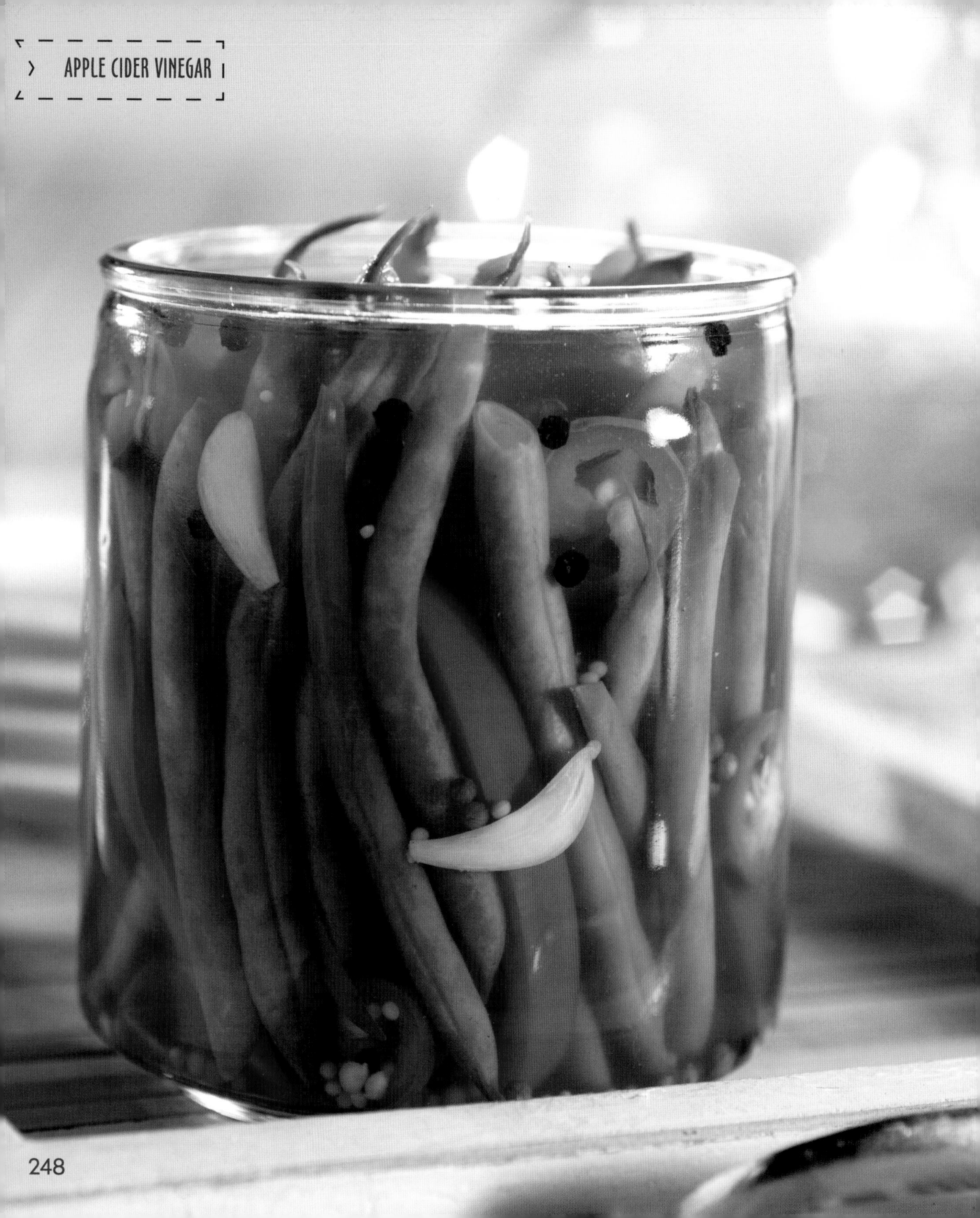

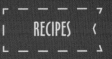

QUICK PICKLED GREEN BEANS
Makes 6 servings

½ pound (3½ cups loosely packed) whole green beans

½ red bell pepper, cut into strips (optional)

1 jalapeño or other hot pepper,* sliced

1 clove garlic, cut in half

1 bay leaf

1 cup white wine vinegar

1 cup water

½ cup white wine

1 tablespoon sugar

1 tablespoon salt

1 tablespoon whole coriander seeds

1 tablespoon mustard seeds

1 tablespoon whole peppercorns

1. Wash beans; remove stem ends, if desired. Place in glass dish just large enough to hold beans and 2½ cups liquid. Add bell pepper strips, if desired. Tuck jalapeño slices, garlic and bay leaf among beans.

2. Combine vinegar, water, wine, sugar, salt, coriander seeds, mustard seeds and peppercorns in medium saucepan. Bring to a boil, stirring until sugar and salt are dissolved. Reduce heat to low; simmer 5 minutes.

3. Pour mixture over beans, making sure beans are fully submerged in liquid. If not, add additional hot water to cover. Cover and refrigerate at least 24 hours.**

4. Drain beans. Remove and discard bay leaf.

*Chile peppers can sting and irritate the skin, so wear rubber gloves when handling peppers and do not touch your eyes.

**The flavor is best after 48 hours. The beans can be stored in the refrigerator for up to five days.

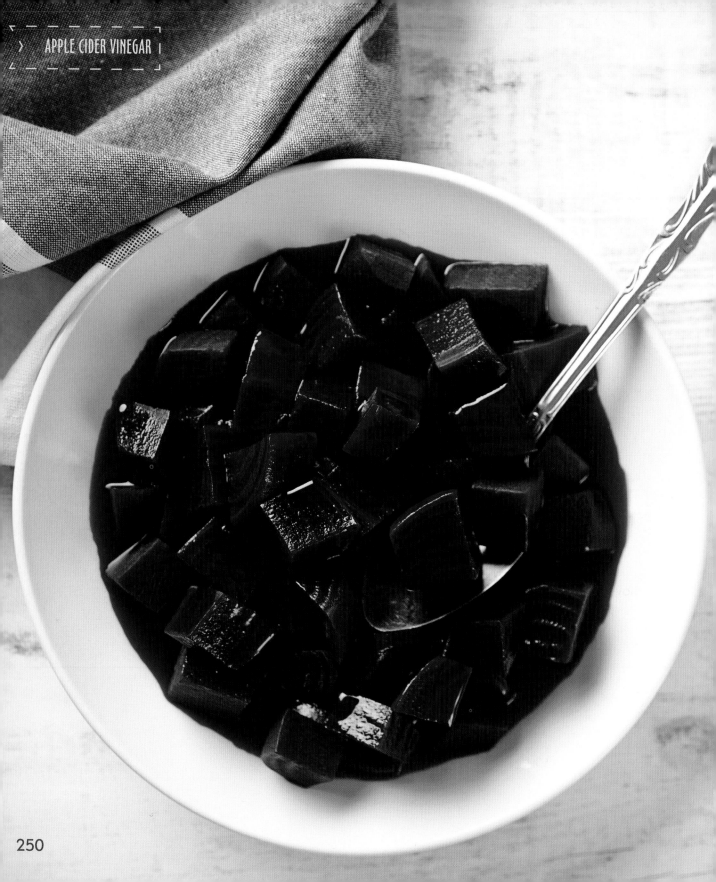

HARVARD BEETS
Makes 6 servings

~~~~~~

- 2 pounds fresh beets, peeled and cut into 1-inch cubes
- ⅔ cup sugar
- ½ cup apple cider vinegar
- ¼ cup water
- 1 teaspoon salt
- 1 tablespoon cornstarch
- 2 tablespoons butter

SLOW COOKER DIRECTIONS:

1. Place beets in slow cooker. Add sugar, vinegar, water and salt; stir to blend. Cover; cook on HIGH 3 hours or until beets are just tender.

2. Remove 2 tablespoons juice from slow cooker to small bowl. Stir cornstarch into juice until smooth; whisk into slow cooker. Stir in butter. Cover; cook on HIGH 30 minutes.

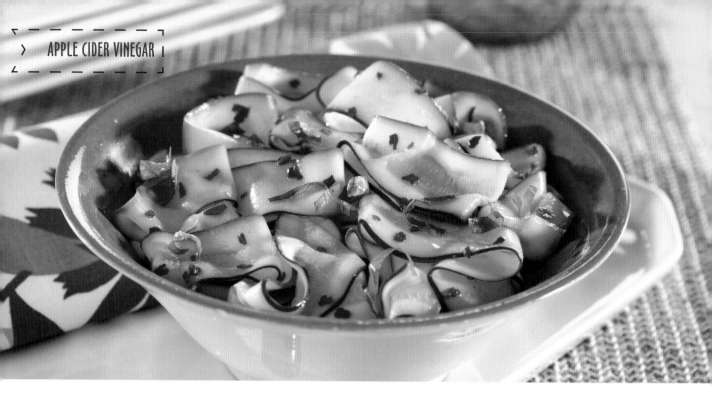

HERBED ZUCCHINI RIBBONS
Makes 4 servings

- 3 small zucchini (about ¾ pound total)
- 2 tablespoons olive oil
- 1 tablespoon white wine vinegar
- 2 teaspoons chopped fresh basil leaves
   or ½ teaspoon dried basil
- ½ teaspoon red pepper flakes
- ¼ teaspoon ground coriander
   Salt and black pepper

1. To make zucchini ribbons, cut tip and stem ends from zucchini with paring knife. Using vegetable peeler, begin at stem end and make continuous ribbons down length of each zucchini.

2. To steam zucchini ribbons, place steamer basket in large saucepan; add 1 inch of water. (Water should not touch bottom of basket.) Place zucchini ribbons in steamer basket; cover. Bring to a boil over high heat. When pan begins to steam, check zucchini for doneness. (It should be crisp-tender.) Transfer zucchini to warm serving dish with slotted spatula or tongs.

3. Combine oil, vinegar, basil, red pepper and coriander in small glass bowl, whisking until oil is thoroughly blended.

4. Pour dressing mixture over zucchini ribbons; toss gently to coat. Season with salt and black pepper. Serve immediately or refrigerate up to 2 days.

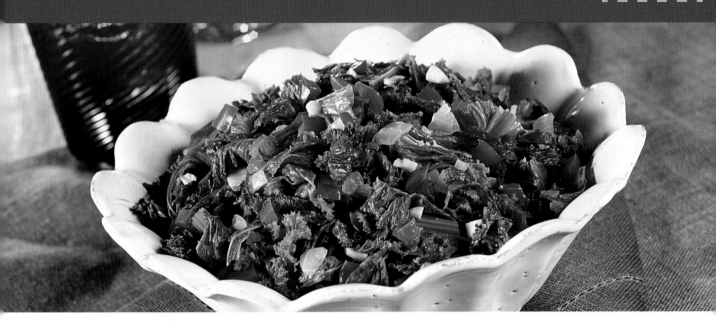

GARLICKY MUSTARD GREENS
Makes 4 servings

- 2 pounds mustard greens
- 1 teaspoon olive oil
- 1 cup chopped onion
- 2 cloves garlic, minced
- ¾ cup chopped red bell pepper
- ½ cup chicken or vegetable broth
- 1 tablespoon apple cider vinegar
- 1 teaspoon sugar

1. Remove stems and any wilted leaves from greens. Stack several leaves; roll up. Cut crosswise into 1-inch slices. Repeat with remaining greens.

2. Heat oil in large saucepan over medium heat. Add onion and garlic; cook and stir 5 minutes or until onion is tender. Stir in greens, bell pepper and broth. Reduce heat to low. Cook, covered, 25 minutes or until greens are tender, stirring occasionally.

3. Combine vinegar and sugar in small bowl; stir until sugar dissolves. Stir into cooked greens; remove from heat. Serve immediately.

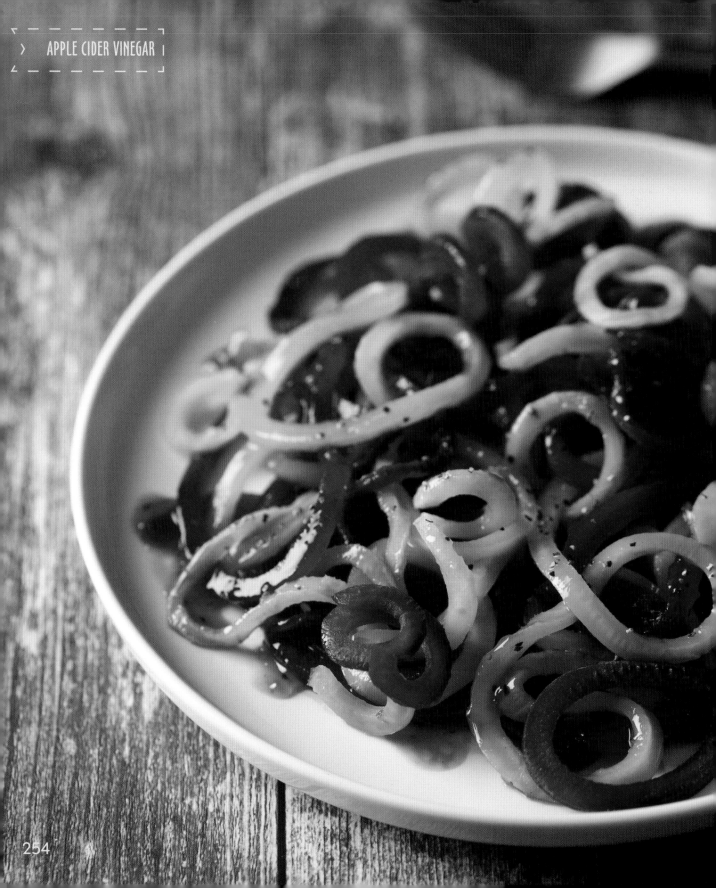

HONEYED BEETS
Makes 4 servings

~~~~~~~~~~~~~~~~~~~~~

- 1   medium red beet (8 ounces)
- 1   medium golden beet (8 ounces)
- 1   tablespoon vegetable oil
- ¼   cup unsweetened apple juice
- 2   tablespoons apple cider vinegar
- 1   tablespoon honey
- 2   teaspoons cornstarch
     Salt and black pepper

1. Preheat oven to 425°F. Line baking sheet with parchment paper.

2. Spiral beets with fine spiral blade; cut into desired lengths. Spread on prepared baking sheet, keeping golden beets separate from red beets; drizzle with oil. Bake 15 minutes or until tender, stirring occasionally.

3. Combine apple juice, vinegar, honey and cornstarch in large saucepan; cook over medium heat 8 to 10 minutes or until shimmering, stirring occasionally. Stir in beets; season to taste with salt and pepper. Simmer 3 minutes or until glazed.

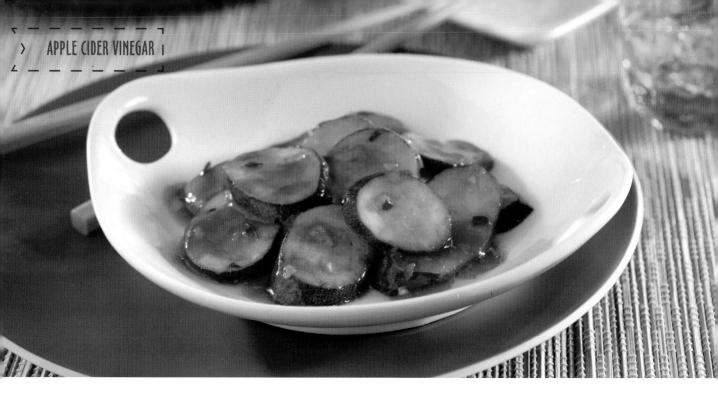

HOT AND SOUR ZUCCHINI

Makes 4 servings

- 2 teaspoons minced fresh ginger
- 1 clove garlic, minced
- ¼ teaspoon red pepper flakes or crushed Szechuan peppercorns
- 1 pound zucchini, cut into ¼-inch slices
- 2 teaspoons sugar
- 1 teaspoon cornstarch
- 2 tablespoons red wine vinegar
- 2 tablespoons soy sauce
- 1 tablespoon peanut or vegetable oil
- 1 teaspoon dark sesame oil

1. Combine ginger, garlic and red pepper flakes in small bowl. Add zucchini; toss to coat.

2. Combine sugar and cornstarch in small bowl. Stir in vinegar and soy sauce until smooth.

3. Heat peanut oil in large skillet over medium-high heat. Add zucchini mixture; cook and stir 4 to 5 minutes or until zucchini is crisp-tender.

4. Stir vinegar mixture. Add to skillet; cook 15 seconds or until sauce boils and thickens. Stir in sesame oil.